ALL
THE PROOF

Everything about the prostate, its disorders and treatments

It's natural, it's my health

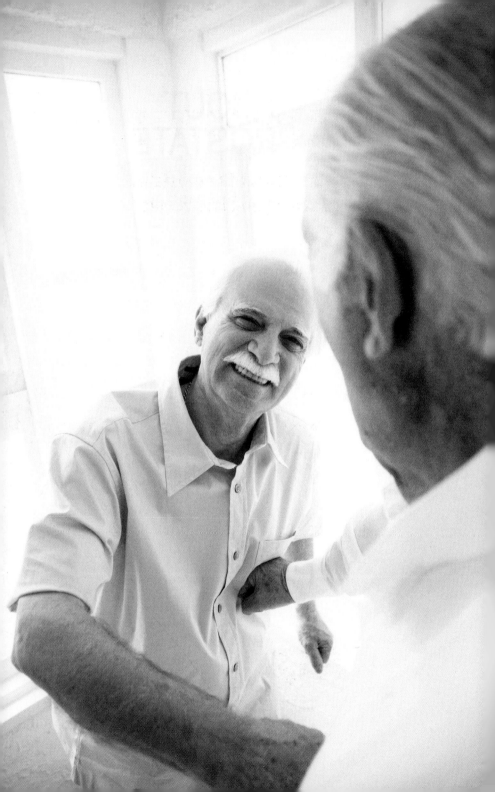

ALL ABOUT THE PROSTATE

Everything about the prostate, its disorders and treatments

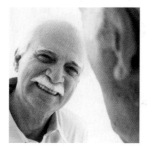

Dr Patrice Pfeifer

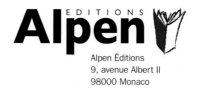

Alpen Éditions
9, avenue Albert II
98000 Monaco

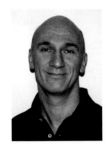

Dr.Patrice Pfeifer is a urologist in Limoges and member of the French Urologist Association. A prostate specialist, our book is the result of fifteen years of medical experience.

Exclusive copyrights:
©Alpen Éditions
9, avenue Albert II
98000 Monaco
Tel: +377 97 77 62 10
Fax: +377 97 77 62 11
web: www.alpen.mc

Printed in Italy
ISBN: 978-2-35934-045-7

Introduction

You suffer from prostate problems or you do not have any symptoms, but you have heard talk about the prostate and you wonder about it and ask if you could be affected.

One of your friends has prostate problems although he is in good health and you are worried about yours.

A close relative passed away from prostate cancer: can it be transmitted genetically and are you at a higher risk for getting it?

Are there ways to prevent prostate diseases (diet, healthy lifestyle or sexuality)?

You take medicine for your prostate: should you expect to be operated on someday?

These are the questions men will one day ask themselves when they turn fifty.

Broadcasts and medical articles are multiplying with the development of the media and our society.
"There are more and more prostate cancers, Doctor, why is that?" And if it was simply because there is more and more talk about it, when it was always one of the leading causes of death in men…

They told you that you have a prostate adenoma, and you are afraid that you'll have to be operated on someday or you are worried that it may become malignant…

This book will provide you with explanations so you can better understand the reasons for:

- screening;
- medicine;
- changing your lifestyle;
- simple monitoring;
- interest in an operation;

but also be reassured about your fears that you may feel wrongly about, simply because you didn't dare to speak up. More importantly, this book will help you to live with your prostate, since it will no longer be a taboo subject…

It will encourage you to eat a more balanced diet to prevent certain prostate diseases. It will inform you on these pathologies, help you to ask your doctor more informed questions and better understand what your doctor proposes. However, by no means can this book replace the 7 to 15 years of your family doctor's or urologist's studies, with their experience they are the best to turn to for advice.

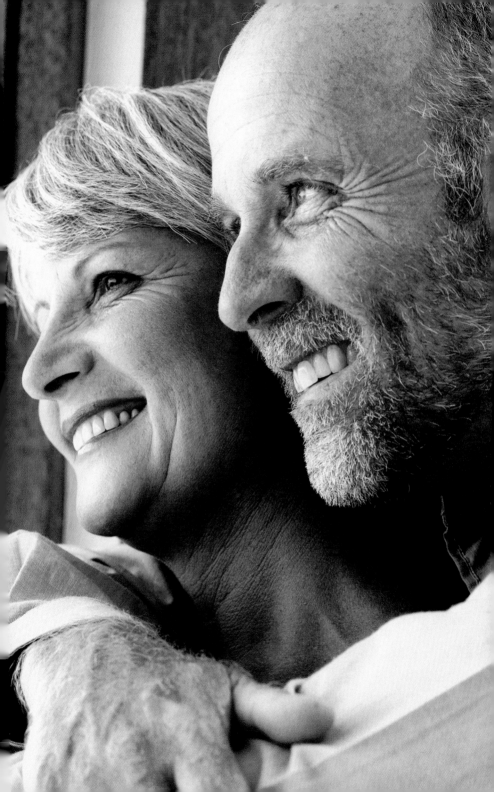

TABLE OF CONTENTS

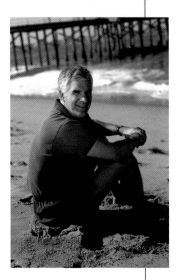

THE PATHS THAT LEAD TO THE PROSTATE

There are many reasons behind a first trip to the urologist, even if you don't have any symptoms.

Just to find out the situation

You are 50-60 years old, you have heard people talk about the prostate and you decide it's time to go to a urologist, just for a check-up.

He will ask you if you have problems urinating and then he will perform a digital rectal exam *(see pg. 22)*. If he detects a suspicious area, he will propose a biopsy. If the digital exam is normal or if your prostate is actually "enlarged" but you urinate normally, he will suggest a follow-up.

He will also prescribe a blood test to measure a protein which indicates the activity of the prostate called PSA *(Prostate Specific Antigen) (see pg. 26)*. He will tell you to contact him if your PSA is high. If it is high, a biopsy may be necessary.

The normal PSA level varies with age	
Your age	**The normal level is** (in nanograms per milliliter)
40-49	< 2.5
50-59	< 3.5
60-69	< 4.5
70-79	< 6.5

An urge to urinate frequently

You have been referred to a urologist by your family doctor because your PSA is above normal or because you have trouble urinating.

The urologist will ask you how many times you get up to urinate at night (up to twice per night is normal), how the force of your urine stream is, and if the urge is pressing, if you are able to hold it without any problems.

He will then perform a digital rectal exam in order to discover the volume and consistency of your prostate.

At this point different cases may occur:

• your prostate is enlarged and flexible, this is an adenoma which will not harm you and requires no treatment;

• your prostate is normal size but the urologist feels a hard, or simply firm area, and proposes biopsies to eliminate an early stage cancer, a stage where you can be cured with a suitable treatment;

• your prostate has a normal size and consistency but your PSA level is high: an early stage cancer is still a fear and the urologist may suggest a new PSA test in a few months or systematic biopsies if you are young (less than 70 years old).

Lastly, he will probably have you do an **endorectal prostate sonogram** to measure the volume of your prostate since the PSA level sometimes increases simply with the size of the prostate even when there is no cancer. In this case, your PSA just needs to be kept under surveillance.

Are you having problems urinating?
Your doctor will talk to you about...

- **pollakiuria** if you urinate more than twice a night and 10 to 15 times a day;
- **urinary urgency**, if the urge to urinate is pressing, sometimes unbearable or even uncontrollable. These manifestations are due to the fact that the prostate is located under the bladder, which is stimulated in some way and contracts too often;
- **dysuria** if you have to wait to urinate. The stream is thin, weak, irregular and sometimes separate. Your urination is long and ends abruptly with a few drips at the end. The compression of the urethra by the prostate causes dysuria often more pronounced in the early hours.

Sometimes there is pain and burning at the end of urinating and painful ejaculation during sexual intercourse.

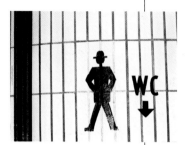

DISORDERS THAT AROUSE SUSPICION

Blood in your urine, burning sensations or even not being able to urinate at all... disorders which are serious to a certain extent and may also involve the prostate.

Where does the blood come from?

All hematurias require a urological examination, including a sonogram, an intravenous urography and bladder cystoscopy to look for other causes of the hematuria (bladder cancer, stones, kidney cancer and ureter cancer).

Urinary tract infections: when the prostate is in the picture

A urinary tract infection requires a complete urology checkup. If the infection is due to prostate hypertrophy, a treatment will be needed for this gland, but if the infections are too frequent, an operation may be the solution.

When there is blood in your urine

A few drops of blood may turn the urine in your bladder red. This is called hematuria. Do not panic because there is no danger. This presence of blood is **more alarming than dangerous.** Drink plenty of water to "flush it out" and call your doctor…

Hematuria may be due to:
- simple enlargement of the prostate;
- a urinary tract infection which "inflames" and weakens the bladder walls, making them bleed;
- bladder stones which irritate the walls.

When the prostate is the cause it usually results in an initial hematuria (the blood comes out first, then the urine gets lighter). These hematurias occur from time to time and are not dangerous. Nevertheless, if they continue they may lead to a decision at some point to operate on the prostate.

You feel a burning sensation during urination

This is probably a urinary tract infection which is causing an irritation of the bladder and urethra. Burning is often coupled with a frequent urge to urinate, even as many as twelve times a night. Since the bladder does not have time to fill again, very little urine comes out each time. Sometimes the irritation is so bad that the bladder may bleed. You may have a temperature (fever of 100 to 104 °F), which usually means that the bacteria has penetrated the prostate (with a risk of septicemia).

The infection is diagnosed with a urine test and quickly **improves with antibiotics.** Treatment lasts three weeks for urinary tract infections accompanied by a temperature.

Acute urinary retention: "urinate or die"

You have not urinated in 24 hours or more, your bladder is full and obstructed: you have an urge to urinate but you can't. Your lower abdomen is bloated, and very painful when pressed. This feeling of roundness, above the pubis is called full bladder: the bladder can contain more than a liter of urine! This is acute urinary retention.

It does not help to try and force it or wait. There is only one thing to do: **insert a catheter** into the urethra canal and empty the bladder. You will get immediate relief. Call your family doctor, or go straight to the emergency room. The catheter is left in for a few days to let the bladder "rest". Once it is pulled out you have a one out of two chance of being able to urinate normally again. But be careful of relapses!

Acute urine retention may turn out to be a prostate hypertrophy, not noticed up to now due to the lack of apparent symptoms. It may also occur in a man already being treated for the prostate; in this case it indicates a turning point in the advancement of the disease. A prostate operation will probably be necessary.

What contributes to urine retention?

- a prolonged effort to retain it;

- certain medicines (medicine for cold and the bronchial tubes and tranquilizers);

- constipation;

- spinal anesthesia (anesthesia to numb the lower part of the body for an operation for something else;

- exaggerated consumption of certain foods and drinks: dinner parties washed down with champagne, white wine, cordials, beer ...

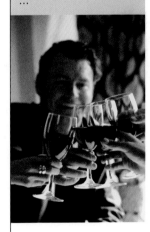

WHAT IS THE PROSTATE?

A bit of regional anatomy

In order to understand the symptoms and repercussions of prostate diseases, you first have to understand how the male urinary tract works.

The prostate is located under the bladder (more precisely under the bladder neck) and around the urethra. It is important not to mix up the urethra which is the canal through which urine is discharged that comes from the bladder and the ureters which are the tubes carrying urine from the kidneys to the bladder. The prostate is composed of three lobes: the right and left lobes and the middle lobe located behind and below the neck of the bladder.

The role of sphincters

The portion located under the bladder is called the prostate base and the other end is the apex, which is situated just before the **striated sphincter** of the urethra. This sphincter is a muscle which ensures voluntary urinary continence. This is what is in charge of retaining urine. A second smooth sphincter is located around the neck of the bladder and functions automatically.

When the prostate is surgically removed, the striated sphincter is maintained and used to retain urine. In some cases, this sphincter may become weak and cause

To monitor the kidneys, monitor creatinine

Creatinine is a substance released from protein metabolism in the body. It is eliminated from the body by the kidneys and can be measured in both the blood and urine. The blood creatinine level is between 8 and 12 mg/l. Measurement of the blood creatinine level (or creatininemia) shows kidney functioning and is now used instead of urea tests. When the blood creatinine level is normal or low, kidney functioning is good. When creatinine is high, it indicates kidney failure.

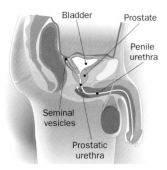

Localization of the prostate

post-op incontinence.

Behind the prostate base are the seminal vesicles, which act as a reservoir for sperm between ejaculations. They are connected to the ejaculatory ducts which cross the prostate to enter the urethra at the *colliculuc seminalis*. These ejaculatory ducts are attached to the prostate and when the gland is completely removed, they must be removed as well. This operation makes the person sterile.

The bladder acts as a reservoir...

The bladder collects the urine produced by the kidneys. It stores urine between two urinations. Its storage capacity depends on its elasticity. Its walls are composed of muscle fibers **(detrusor)**. These fibers stretch as the bladder fills. Once a certain volume is passed, the reflex phenomena reverse the functioning of these fibers and start to contract. This is when you feel an urge to urinate. The striated sphincter (up to this point closed to retain urine) opens and urination occurs. The stream of urine quickly increases in strength and later decreases as the bladder starts to empty.

... and the kidneys as filter

There are two kidneys. They clean the blood of all toxic waste, waste that is later eliminated in the urine. Of these wastes, the best known is urea. An accumulation of urea in the blood means kidney failure. If the urea level is too high it may cause problems with wakefulness and even lead to coma. This is called "uremia".

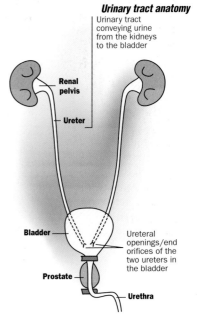

Urinary tract anatomy

Urinary tract conveying urine from the kidneys to the bladder

The prostate: a gland and a muscle at the same time

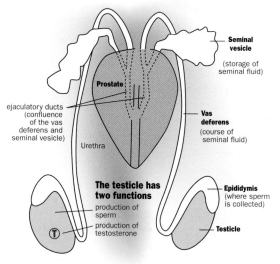

- Seminal vesicle (storage of seminal fluid)
- Prostate
- ejaculatory ducts (confluence of the vas deferens and seminal vesicle)
- Vas deferens (course of seminal fluid)
- Urethra
- **The testicle has two functions**
  - production of sperm
  - production of testosterone
- Epididymis (where sperm is collected)
- Testicle

Muscles and fibers

The prostate is composed of gland, muscle and fiber areas. The gland areas produce secretions and the muscle areas are where contractions start; alpha receptors (which receive the stimulations of a chemical messenger called adrenaline) are located in this muscle region. When these receptors are blocked by medicine called alpha-blockers, the prostate muscle fibers relax, resulting in relaxation of the gland and better urine flow.

The prostate is a small gland, even poorly placed, at a urinary and genital triangle, where the simple mention of it brings to mind aging and diseases which raise fear of a loss of virility.

Like a walnut

The prostate is a small gland, more or less the size of a walnut, and is only found in men. It is used to **produce secretions** which help to produce sperm. That is its only role.

It is not a vital gland (unlike the liver, which is also a gland, but humans can't live without it). So it can be removed in certain circumstances, without any danger to the organism.

Its problems occur due to its anatomical situation that causes its removal to often result in urinary or sexual complications.

When the prostate is diseased

There are three prostate diseases:
• prostatitis or an infection of the prostate;
• benign adenoma or hypertrophy of the prostate, this is the most frequent. This means an enlargement of the prostate. This involves a benign tumor, which means that it is not cancerous (careful: tumor does not mean cancer, but simply an increase in the size of part of an organ);
• cancer, a real curse up to fifteen years ago, has become increasingly easier to control with screening techniques and current treatments. This is a malignant tumor of the prostate, and malignant means cancer.
So, we have two types of prostate tumor:
– one, benign: adenoma
– the other, malignant: cancer.

Central prostate and peripheral prostate

To better understand adenoma and cancer, as well as the symptoms involved, look at the diagram on the side. This drawing shows that the prostate is composed of two parts:
• The central prostate (also called transition area or cranial prostate) surrounds the urinary tract. As it increases in volume, it compresses the urinary tract, making it difficult to discharge urine. Adenoma develops starting from this central prostate. It has nothing to do with cancer and will never become cancerous.
• The peripheral prostate (also called the peripheral area or caudal prostate), surrounds the central prostate. This is where cancer starts, but usually not adenoma.

Diagram of the two prostate areas

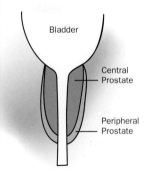

Bladder

Central Prostate

Peripheral Prostate

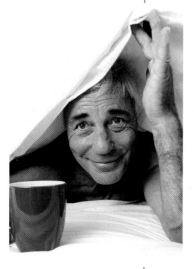

When the prostate acts up

A decrease in urine stream force and frequent nightly trips to the bathroom are signs of a prostate problem. But this can occur even with no symptoms.

The symptoms are related to the enlargement of the gland, but many prostate hypertrophies go totally unnoticed and can only be detected with a digital rectal exam. So, even if you have no problem urinating, this does not mean your prostate is normal.

When the prostate becomes a nuisance

An enlarged prostate causes difficult urination, otherwise related to bladder irritation and compression of the urethra. A study by ANFUC (National Association of Continuous Urologic Education) has made it possible to classify the symptoms based on their frequency.

Symptom frequency for a group of 159 patients

Symptoms	Percentage
Decrease in stream force	90
Nocturnal pollakiuria	87
Daytime pollakiuria	85
Delayed stream	61
Sensation of incomplete urination	55
Urgency	49
Post-void drips	40
Interrupted stream	23

The list could also include time to time pain with urination, burning at the end of urination and painful ejaculation.

Urge to continuously urinate

Pollakiuria refers to when the number of urinations exceeds 2 at night and 5 during the day. The impact of this on daily life may be difficult to cope with. These urges harm the sleep of a couple, disrupt long car trips, professional life (meetings and conferences), spare time (movies and theater), strolling and shopping.

Incontinence is really a false incontinence

Urinary leaking in prostate disorders cannot be compared to incontinence. There are urinary disorders due to prostate hypertrophy: post-void dripping, leaks due to an urge to urinate and "over-flowing" of urine due to chronic retention. They will disappear when the prostate hypertrophy is treated.

Pelvic congestion symptoms

A more or less painful sensation in the pelvis, in the sub-pubic region, perineum, or testes which may be associated to varying degrees with the symptoms described above.

The other symptoms (hematurias, urinary tract infections and acute urinary retention or obstruction) reveal a prostate hypertrophy, but they can occur in men who had not complained of anything up to that point.

Blood in the sperm

When traces of blood are found in the sperm it is referred to as hematospermia. This is fairly frequent and not serious, but it does require a trip to the urologist.

Long term complications

When the prostate becomes too enlarged it is impossible to urinate normally. All of the urinary system becomes progressively affected.

The bladder empties poorly

Prostate hypertrophy negatively affects urine flow and the bladder is forced to fight against the pressure the prostate puts on its walls to discharge the urine. The detrusor (muscle that pushes down and expels urine from the bladder), since it has to work more "develops muscles", it gets thicker and the volume of urine that the bladder can hold decreases a bit at a time. At the same time the urge to urinate becomes more and more frequent. Over time, the detrusor becomes "worn out" and the bladder no longer empties completely: this is referred to as post-void residual.

The constant presence of urine in the bladder can lead to urinary tract infections.

This residual increases progressively, the bladder empties less and less and becomes bloated.

Undesirable stones

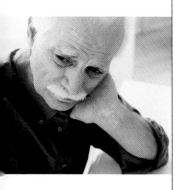

The urine which stagnates in the bladder and urinary tract infections can cause the formation of stones in the bladder. This is called a "stone disease". The presence of these stones is not connected in any way to kidney stones. Bladder stones originate and grow in the bladder. They can be numerous and reach the size of a quail egg. If they irritate the bladder walls, they can cause bleeding. If there are too many of them, an operation on the bladder can be performed to remove them. So the prostate is operated on because it is the source of stone formation.

Chronic retention

Over time the bloating of the bladder becomes worse and worse. It does not contract as well, and there is less urge to urinate. The bladder is almost always full, at times with more than a pint of urine. When it overflows, this is referred to as false overflow incontinence.

Careful of danger to kidneys

At this stage if nothing is done, the bloating goes to the next stage. The bladder empties poorly; plus the ureters discharge increasingly poorly and bloat, and then it is the turn of the renal pelvises and calices. Then the urine starts to stagnate in the kidneys: there is a threat of kidney failure. This generally only appears after many years of neglected urinary tract disorders and has minor symptoms: nausea, difficulty with bowel movements, fatigue and problems with wakefulness, even leading to coma. Kidney functioning becomes gradually worse, starting with kidney failure which is reversible if the prostate disorder is treated. If it is neglected, the affliction is irreversible. This situation, which requires dialysis, is thankfully becoming rarer and rarer.

With an untreated prostate the entire urinary tract suffers

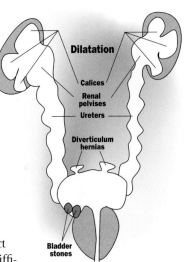

Dilatation

Calices

Renal pelvises

Ureters

Diverticulum hernias

Bladder stones

Corners in the bladder

As the detrusor thickens, certain areas become weaker and the bladder mucous membrane forms small "hernias" called diverticulum in this spot. These diverticulum hernias contain and sometimes retain urine, giving rise to urinary tract infections here as well. Their association with a thickening of the bladder wall gives them an appearance of a "trabeculated bladder".

SEEING A UROLOGIST
Digital rectal exam

The prostate is located at the level of the perineum, just behind the rectum, so there is only one way to examine it: with a digital rectal exam.

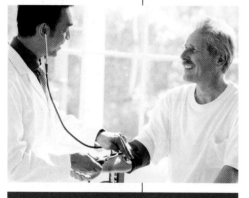

The prostate enlarges with age

a few grams at birth;

around 15 to 20 grams between 25 and 40 years old;

if hypertrophied, it can reach 100 to 300 grams and even more.

How the exam is done?

Your doctor will ask you to get into one of the following positions:

- on your back, in "gynecological" position;
- on your hands and knees, in "crawling" position;
lying on your left side, with legs bent in a curled up position;
- in a standing position, with your trunk bent slightly forward. This technique is practiced on older men, who are not very alert and have trouble getting up on the examining table. A finger is introduced into the rectum and the entire surface of the prostate can be felt immediately. The doctor uses a plastic glove and Vaseline to introduce his finger into the anus to evaluate the surface of the prostate. If he does this gently this exam is not painful, except in exceptional cases with a contracted or narrow anus.

This exam is essential for getting an idea of the size and condition of the prostate. Some men try to avoid it: "But doctor, my blood test for the prostate was normal!" So I explain to them that they can have prostate cancer with a normal PSA and that only a digital rectal exam makes it possible to diagnose it.

Next, they tell me: "But Doctor, you could look at it with a sonogram on my stomach, like they do for pregnant women!". I explain to them that it would be like looking at the prostate at the end of a hallway, in the dark and with a poor telescope!

Why is this exam necessary?

A digital rectal exam makes it possible to discover three fundamental parameters:

• **the size of the prostate:** urologists often express this in grams and thanks to the digital rectal exam, they can tell you "your prostate is around 30, 50 or 100 grams…". The measurement of the size is later refined by sonogram.

• **Consistency:** this is an essential parameter. If the prostate is hypertrophied but still supple, the tumor is most likely benign (except in some cases which will be rescreened with PSA). A hard area or a hard prostate generally indicates cancer.

• **Sensitivity:** a prostate with adenoma or cancer is not painful, at most there will be an unpleasant feeling of an urge to urinate during the digital rectal exam. On the other hand, an infected prostate (prostatitis) is extremely painful.

After age 50, an exam every year

The digital rectal exam is the surest way of screening and the best prostate examination method and best way for discovering a tumor, adenoma or cancer. This exam needs to be done annually and systematically after age 50.

No false modesty

The digital rectal exam is the only way to get to the prostate and you need to learn to put your "false modesty" aside. The digital rectal exam is not a degrading exam for men, and it makes it possible to save lives by discovering cancer at an early stage when it can be cured.

Sonogram

Harmless, it is often done during the first check-up and is used to establish a first "ID card" of the prostate and urinary tract to use for future comparison.

Prostate sonogram

The prostate sonogram is performed by inserting a tube in the anus.

This exam is generally not painful. It supplements the information from the digital rectal exam and is thus always associated with it. It is called "the eye at the tip of the urologist's finger".

The sonogram is used to:

• precisely measure the volume of the prostate (in cm^3 or grams). This is useful for interpreting the PSA level or for selecting a surgical technique before operating on an adenoma;

• detecting "dubious" areas which require a biopsy *(see box)*.

Prostate sonogram in practice

An endorectal sonogram of the prostate is performed at the urologist's or at a radiologist's. Lying on one side, the doctor will gently insert a sonogram probe the size of a finger into your anus. Insertion of the probe is made easier by using a gel. The image is obtained using ultrasound and not X rays. The image is used to study your prostate up close.

The urinary tract from every angle

The bladder needs to be full at the time of the exam. The urologist will spread gel on the abdomen (just like for pregnant women!) before placing the sonogram probe.

The image lets the doctor discover:

• the condition of the bladder: presence of stones, possible tumor, general appearance (trabeculated bladder) and post-void residual;
• the approximate size of the prostate;
• condition of the kidneys with possible dilatation of its cavities which may be a side effect of prostate hypertrophy.

The process for a complete exam

The patient needs to drink a quart of water an hour before the exam so that his bladder is full.
• First on the back: sonogram exam of the two kidneys and then bladder.
• Then on the left side: digital rectal exam followed by endorectal sonogram.
• Urination in the urinary output tester.
• New bladder sonogram to measure the post-void residual.

A technique discovered at the beginning of the 1950's

In 1953 Dr. John Wild and the engineer John Reid created the first sonogram of breast cancer in Minneapolis. This is the principle of submarine sonars applied to the human body! A probe emits sound waves in the direction of the organs to observe. The waves are reflected based on the density of the tissue encountered, making it possible to obtain a precise image of the condition of the various tissues.

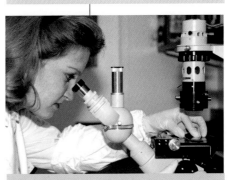

Biopsy: an essential analysis

This is the only exam that can confirm a cancer diagnosis. Most often it is an adenocarcinoma. The anatomy-pathology lab, will also indicate the degree of aggressiveness of the tumor using the "Gleason score" ranging from 2 to 10. The higher the number, the more dangerous the tumor.

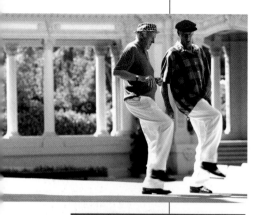

PSA: the prostate's health rating

The level of PSA (*prostate specific antigen*) in the blood is an essential parameter for screening and monitoring prostate diseases.

PSA level based on age

Age range	Normal PSA rates (in ng/ml)
40 - 49	< 2.5
50 - 59	< 3.5
60 - 69	< 4.5
70 - 79	< 6.5

A specific protein

The prostate specific antigen is a protein produced by the prostate and present in the blood. It is specific to the prostate, which means that no other organ produces it. Thus it is only present in men.

This protein is measured in the blood, and it is not necessary to have an empty stomach at the time of the test.

PSA is not a toxic compound for the body, and in itself is not dangerous. Having a slightly raised level of PSA after age 50, without any other problems does not require treatment. A high PSA level cannot be compared with, say, a high cholesterol level: the latter definitely represents a risk factor for cardiovascular diseases. It is different for PSA. It is not the PSA in itself that needs to be treated. It is simply a sign that should drive you to consult your urologist.

How is PSA interpreted?

The normal level varies based on the test methods: it is less than 2.5 or 4 ng/l. It increases spontaneously with age and is also correlated to the volume of the prostate. Thus a PSA less than or equal to 4 ng/ml does not necessarily mean that the prostate is normal and a slightly high PSA between 4 and 10 ng/ml does not necessarily mean cancer. PSA is specific to the prostate and not to a particular prostate disease and this is the problem. Thus, to be interpreted correctly it needs to be combined with a digital rectal exam and a prostate sonogram. By taking into account all this data, your urologist will be able to make a diagnosis. If the PSA is disproportionately high compared to the prostate volume, most likely a biopsy will be needed. At an equal volume, a gram of prostate cancer cells secretes 10 times more PSA than a gram of prostate adenoma.

Adenoma or cancer?

Other parameters can help the urologist make a diagnosis.

• **PSA velocity**
This involves tracking the evolution of PSA over time. Blood tests are taken at regular intervals, every three or six months. The test is always analyzed in the same lab so that the results can be compared.
If the PSA increases with each test, most likely cancer is involved. In this case a biopsy is necessary.

• **PSA density**
This is the PSA level compared to the prostate volume evaluated by endorectal sonogram. There is a theoretical density above which there is a risk of cancer. However, this interpretation method is only used on a case by case basis.

What causes PSA to rise

prostatitis
prostate adenoma
prostate cancer
urinary tract infection
acute urinary retention
digital rectal exam
prostate biopsy

Measuring free PSA

The PSA discussed to this point is the total PSA. We now know that free PSA (part of the total PSA which is not associated with proteins) exists in the blood. In the case of cancer, the free PSA rate is weaker than in the case of prostate adenoma. Thus it becomes interesting to calculate the ratio of free PSA to total PSA. If the obtained figure is less than 20% (or 15% based on the lab) this means there is a risk of cancer. Your urologist will certainly want a biopsy.

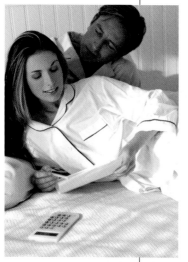

Calculate your symptom score

In order to evaluate your problem and the impact of your urinary disorder on your everyday life, some urologists will have you fill out a questionnaire to calculate your international prostatic symptom score (IPSS).

For each question enter the best answer and total your points in the two tables.

The first figure gives an indication of the intensity of the symptoms (from 0 to 35), the second the amount of perceived bother (from 1 to 6).

How does the urologist use this score?

Let's say, on your first trip to the urologist your score is S15Q5. After treatment, if it becomes S3Q1, the medicine is very effective, and treatment can be continued. If it becomes S13Q4, the medicine is not acting, and another treatment method will have to be set up.

Sperm in the urine?

A whitish, milky appearing liquid, may mix with the urine. This is not sperm. These are secretions from small glands located around the urethra (paraurethra glands). This phenomenon is called urethral discharge and is not serious or cause for alarm.

Can urinary disorders be psychological?

Stress and anxiety can cause an urge to urinate frequently. Often, these frequent urges are accompanied by a weak urine stream, due to poor opening of the neck of the bladder. Insomnia can also be responsible for frequent nighttime urination.

* IPSS : International Prostatic Symptom Score

1 - Over the past month, how often have you had a sensation of not emptying your bladder completely after you finished urinating?

not at all	less than 20% of the time	less than half the time	about half the time	more than half the time	almost always
0	1	2	3	4	5

2 - Over the past month, how often have you had to urinate again less than 2 hours after you finished urinating?

not at all	less than 20% of the time	less than half the time	about half the time	more than half the time	almost always
0	1	2	3	4	5

3 - Over the past month, how often have you stopped and started again several times when you urinated?

not at all	less than 20% of the time	less than half the time	about half the time	more than half the time	almost always
0	1	2	3	4	5

4 - Over the past month, how often have you found it difficult to postpone urination?

not at all	less than 20% of the time	less than half the time	about half the time	more than half the time	almost always
0	1	2	3	4	5

5 - Over the past month, how often have you had a weak urinary stream?

not at all	less than 20% of the time	less than half the time	about half the time	more than half the time	almost always
0	1	2	3	4	5

6 - Over the past month, how often have you had to push or strain to begin urination?

not at all	less than 20% of the time	less than half the time	about half the time	more than half the time	almost always
0	1	2	3	4	5

7 - Over the past month how many times did you typically get up to urinate from the time you went to bed at night until the time you got up in the morning?

not at all	less than 20% of the time	less than half the time	about half the time	more than half the time	almost always
0	1	2	3	4	5

◆ Total symptom score **S** =

Quality of life related to urinary symptoms

You have just described how you urinate. If you had to live the rest of your life this way, how would you describe it:

Very satisfying	Satisfying	Fairly satisfying	Half and half	Fairly bothersome	Bothersome	Very bothersome
0	1	2	3	4	5	6

◆ Quality of Life **Q** =

PROSTATE DISORDERS

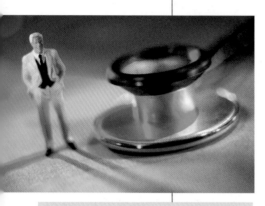

Benign prostatic hypertrophy

One fifty year old man out of five has a prostate disorder. But what happens at that age?

Caucasians more afflicted than Asians

In Western countries, BPH develops in 10% of men starting at age 30, 50% of them starting at age 50 and affects practically all men 80 and older.

Whereas, it is a rare disease in Asian countries.

After age 50 the prostate often starts to get bigger: the cells multiply and form a benign tumor called adenoma: this is benign prostatic hypertrophy (BPH). BPH develops in the central prostate. This hypertrophy involves all three prostate tissues: glandular (adenoma), fibrous (fibroma) and muscular (myoma) thus creating a fibromyomadenoma. An equivalent phenomenon occurs with fibromas in women's uteruses. BPH is not cancerous, nor does it degenerate into cancer. However, it is possible to find cancerous cells in prostatic adenomas. So, the two diseases are associated, but an adenoma never transforms into cancer.

The role of hormones... still a mystery

What are the causes for this disease? It's hard to know exactly. The role of male hormones (androgens) is unquestionable since BPH does not exist in males castrated before puberty and it can disappear after castration. How does androgen intervene? What is the starting process? Many of these questions still remain unanswered. However, researchers are following various leads.

High concentrations of dihydrotestosterone (DHT) are found inside BPH cells, which result from the transformation of testosterone by an enzyme: 5-alpha-reductase. After a certain age, DHT contributes to an excessive development of cells, leading to hypertrophy of the gland.

Other studies implicate female hormones (estrogens). But a hormone hypothesis alone does not explain everything.

Growth factors

Related to androgen hormones (male), "growth factors" called IGF *(insulin-like growth factors)* also seem to play an essential role. They are secreted by certain prostate cells and act mainly on the multiplication, differentiation and survival of the cells. Many growth factors exist, but the reasons that they change in men starting at a certain age is unknown.

Is there a connection with sexual activity?

Unlike what some believe, prostate enlargement has no relation to the frequency of sexual relations. Over the centuries, prostate disorders have been linked to a dissolute sexual life (connected with venereal diseases) as well as abstinence which caused a so-called "enlargement". These are just old wives tales.

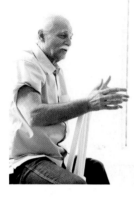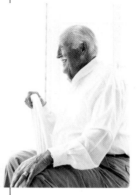

How the disease evolves

A benign prostate tumor develops gradually over many years.

A bigger and bigger prostate

A prostatic hypertrophy starts out microscopic and then becomes macroscopic, i.e. can be felt during a digital rectal exam. The size of the BPH increases regularly over time and can double in volume in a dozen years. It is important to note that there is no direct link between the prostate size and presence or even intensity of urinary disorders. In other words, if your prostate is enlarged this does not necessarily mean you will end up having difficulty urinating.

A high number of BPH have no symptoms. It is possi-

Everyone does not suffer

The increase in prostate volume does not always cause a problem. According to an American study, one man out of two before age 60 who suffers from BPH, says they are handicapped by the disorder: 14% of forty year olds and 24% of fifty year olds. After age 60, 43% say they are bothered by the symptoms.

Monitoring is not treating

Only BPH with symptoms is treated. Actually, why treat something that is not causing any harm? However, some men ask to be treated because they do not accept monitoring very well or even because they are afraid of having an obstruction one day. The treatments do not stop the evolution of the adenoma. The medicines are only there to relieve the symptoms, just like surgery.

ble to have a slightly enlarged prostate, around 20 to 30 grams, with intense, disabling disorders, and a very enlarged prostate of around 300 grams with minimal problems.

Evolution of urinary disorders

The symptoms fluctuate, with periods of worsening or spontaneous improvement, but overall the disorders tend to worsen with time.

Urinary disorders vary with diet, drinks, physical activity and season. They are worse in fall and winter.

BPH: not really a disease

The prostate adenoma is a consequence of age. As long as the prostate, even if enlarged, remains supple, BPH just requires simple monitoring *(see box)*. A check-up will be proposed every other year between age 50 and 60 and then every year after age 60. These examinations make it possible to track the evolution of the adenoma and detect the appearance of any complications. It will also make it possible to screen for early prostate cancer. This monitoring can be recommended for men whose symptoms are light and without particular repercussions on their social life. In this situation, it is possible to simply "make do" by observing some healthy lifestyle rules. This is not a treatment per se, it is simply living in harmony with some minor urinary disorders.

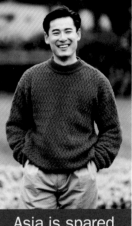

Asia is spared

An estimated 20 million Europeans and more than 7 million Americans suffer from benign prostatic hypertrophy. But autopsies practiced in China over a period of 41 years have shown that BPH affects 6.6% of those of Chinese extraction and 47% of the other ethnic groups. However, the Chinese who emigrate to Western countries are no longer protected, which suggests that environmental and dietetic factors play a role.

BPH risk factors

Epidemiology studies have made it possible to establish a link between certain dietary habits and this prostate disease. Let's see what actual conclusions we can come to.

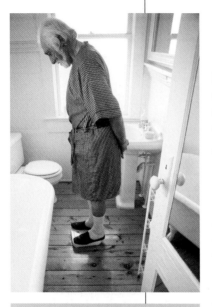

Measure… your health!

Your body mass index (BMI) is obtained by dividing your weight (lb) by your height squared (in²) and multiplying by 703. You are thin if your BMI is between 18.5 and 24. The BMI definitely changes with age, but when over 25, a person is considered overweight, and obese if the BMI exceeds 30. So calculate yours!

The virtues of frugality

By following the diet of several thousand men over years, researchers have been able to identify the diets which contribute to or protect against certain diseases. Various prospective studies of this type have shown that men who have the highest calorie intakes suffer more frequently from benign prostate diseases then "light eaters". The most recent to date, published in April 2002 by the team of Professor Walter Willett of Harvard University, studied 33,344 American men aged 40 to 75 for 8 years. The men who ate an average of 2,700 calories had a 30% higher risk of getting benign prostatic hypertrophy than those who consumed around 1,200 per day. However, alcohol was not counted! The risk of urinary disorders related to prostate dysfunctioning increases 43% in heavy eaters. Do certain foods increase the risk of BPH? The results which are currently available do not make it possible to make a decision.

Tighten your belt!

In a study published in 1994 in the *American Journal of Epidemiology*, researchers at Harvard University showed that men who had a prominent stomach had a higher risk of suffering from prostate diseases than others. They studied 25,892 men aged 40 to 75 from 1987 to 1992. After weighing and measuring them (height and even more importantly waist) the results showed that abdominal fat represents a real risk factor. Men who had a waist bigger than 43 inches have an almost two and a half higher risk of suffering from benign prostatic hypertrophy than those who have a waist under 35 inches.

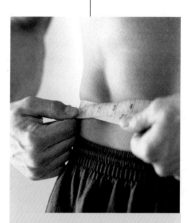

The waist is vital

Another indicator of health is your waist. An American study on 9,000 people in good health aged 20 to 90 evaluated the risk of heart attack based on waist size. A waist size greater than 38.4 inches for men and 34.4 inches for women is associated with a higher cardio-vascular risk.

How many calories a day?

Men (155 pounds)	Inactive	Regular exercise	Sustained sports	Very intense physical activity
20 – 39 years	2 400	2 700	3 080	3 400
40 – 59 years	2 250	2 500	2 900	3 400
60 years and older	around 16 calories per pound of body weight			

Prostate cancer

This is the most frequent cancer in men over age 50 and is the second cause of cancer death in men after lung cancer. The American Cancer Socity estimates that about 218,890 new cases will be diagnosed in the US in 2007 and about 27,050 men will die of the disease.

A Western cancer

The prostate cancer rate is roughly the same in most industrialized countries where life expectancy is long. This cancer mainly affects older men (73 is the average age in a range that goes from 45 to 85) and with the increasing aging of the population thanks to progresses in medicine, its rate is destined to continue to rise. **It affects:**
– 30% of men between 50 and 60;
– 40% of men over 70;
– 70 % of men over 80.
Basically, young men are treated and those over age 80 are closely monitored since they can live for many years with a cancer that advances little or not at all.

Currently, in the United States over 200,000 new cases are diagnosed each year. In the late 1980's the incidence rate of prostate cancer rose dramatically. This increase was due to the growing age of the population, increase in life expectancy and also better screening. Since the early 1990's, however, prostate cancer incidence and mortality in the U.S. have been declining.

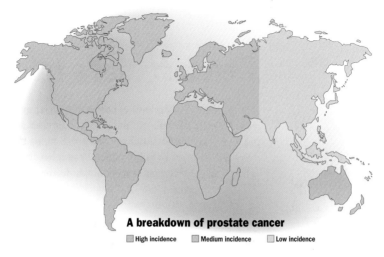

A breakdown of prostate cancer

High incidence   Medium incidence   Low incidence

Heredity is a determinant factor

Heredity plays a predominant role. The risk of developing prostate cancer is doubled if a father, uncle or brother has it. This risk is multiplied by 11 if three relatives are afflicted. Some familial forms appear around age 40 and require early screening in at risk subjects. The localization of the genes responsible for predisposition to prostate cancer has not been clearly established yet.

A hormone-dependent cancer

The more you age, the more you are at risk for prostate cancer. The absence of male hormones protects against the cancer since it does not occur in castrated men. On the contrary, treatment with male hormones is likely to contribute to the development of a pre-existing prostate cancer.

Race and environment...

This cancer is more frequent in Westerners than Asians. But Asians who go to live in the United States have a prostate cancer risk which is 5 times higher, demonstrating that diet plays a role.

African Americans have the highest rate of prostate cancer in the world, pointing to a possible race predisposition.

Cancer: diet's role

Evaluating the effective-
ness of a treatment or
the role of a food is not
an easy thing

Various difficulties occur in carrying out
studies:
- establishing homogenous groups of indi-
viduals which are large enough to be
statistically significant.
- The duration of prostate cancer evolution extends over several years, so monitoring and thus the influence of a food or
treatment, regardless of what it is, requires a minimum of 5 or even 10 years, a
period which is long enough for other
elements to interfere. It is sometimes
even difficult, with major statistical
studies, to say if surgery or radiation
therapy shows the best long-term
improvement and this difficulty is even
greater for the role of diet. So what
remains is just to take the advice that
can be given in this regard to achieve a
healthier lifestyle, and diet rules based
on Asian dietary habits where the incidence of prostate cancer is much lower.

Certain eating habits are not considered as
at risk practices. It is important to understand that this does not mean that it is
"bad" to eat certain foods, but to show that
excessive consumption of certain foods may
play a role in the onset of the disease.

Too many calories

Just like for prostatic hypertrophy, studies
show that men who are affected by
prostate cancer are also those with a diet
too rich in calories. An excessive intake of
energy puts the body in a stimulated state.
Numerous functions stimulated in this
way are involved in the mechanisms for
developing cancer, mainly in terms of cell
proliferation.

Fats

Fats are an important part of the diet and
should ideally represent from 30 to 35% of
daily calorie intake. In the case of prostate
cancer, it seems that a diet high in fat may
contribute to the onset of the disease.
Among the different types of fat, the studies have pinpointed animal fats as the
culprits. By comparing a group with the
disease with a group of healthy men, researchers have
found many times that those who ate more animal fat
had a higher risk of cancer than the others.

Red meat

An American study conducted by Healthcare Professionals on 51,529 men starting in 1986 made it possible to show that men who consume more red meat have a 2 times greater risk of prostate cancer than those who consume less. Cold cuts are also associated with this at risk food class.

Milk

To date, 12 prospective studies on prostate risk factors have shown that the biggest consumers of dairy products have 1.5 to 5.5 times higher risk of getting prostate cancer than those who relinquish these products. In addition, the countries with the highest consumers of dairy products, like the United States, Finland or Sweden also have the highest rates of prostate cancer. It seems that the negative effect of milk is due to calcium which, by reducing the level of a cancer fighting vitamin (vitamin D), contributes to the development of prostate cancer. A study published in 2001 showed that men with a dairy source calcium intake greater than 600 mg per day have a 32% higher risk of getting prostate cancer than those who consume less than 150 mg a day.

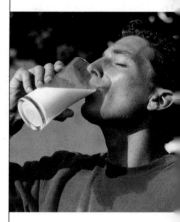

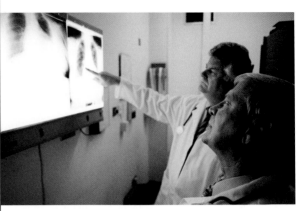

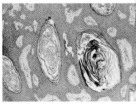

A prostate biopsy is the key to diagnosing cancer. This entails an examination of a prostate specimen under the microscope.

The biology of cancer

A chronic disease, cancer evolves slowly over the years.

A disease which spreads

Cancer starts out in a "cellular" microscopic stage. The cells reproduce until they form a lump which can be felt during a digital rectal exam. **This lump then enlarges and spreads** in the prostate. At this stage it remains localized in the prostate gland. Next, it goes past its limits and spreads more and more, first piercing the capsule, then entering the seminal vesicles, sphincters and bladder. Through the lymph vessels, it will localize in the pelvis ganglion and then the whole organism. The cancer cells can also escape from the blood vessels and fix themselves on other organs, basically the bones, but also the lungs, brain and liver.

So cancer has various evolutionary stages:
• the localized stage when it can still be cured;
• the locally advanced stage where it has gone beyond the limits of the prostate;
• the advanced stage with ganglion or bone metastases most of the time *(see box)*.

Act as early as possible

To be able to recover from prostate cancer, **it must be diagnosed early**, when it is not very developed. If the cancer cells have already invaded all or almost all of the gland, the risk of metastases is already high. Likewise, if the cancer originates at a very small level, the metastasis starts out invisibly. Thus a large cancerous lump localized in the prostate can already have sent cancer cells in the organism. This explains why, even if the prostate has been removed, metastases can develop all the same over subsequent years.

To recover from localized prostate cancer, it needs to be small, thus detectable during a digital rectal exam in the form of a small lump, or so small that it cannot be detected and is revealed by a slight rise in PSA.

However, the higher the PSA reading, the more cancer cells are developing. For the best chances of recovery, the PSA should not have exceeded around 10 ng/ml.

All of this clearly shows one thing: to get prostate cancer at a sufficiently early stage, it must be small, at that point there will be no urinary disorder and the PSA must not be too high: in short, when the man appears to be in good health!

What is a metastasis?

A metastasis is a cancer cell originating from a primary tumor in an organ (or tissue) which migrates to another organ (or tissue) located at a distance, causing the reproduction of a similar lesion. Metastatic transfer is a phenomenon characteristic of the evolution of cancer and malignancy. This spreading corresponds to a cascade of events: invasion of tissues around the tumor, penetration of the blood or lymph vessels, migration, then stopping and formation of a new colony, with escaping from the organism's defense mechanisms.

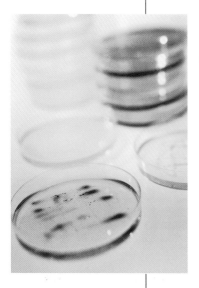

Tracking cancer

In the early stage of cancer a digital rectal exam and PSA provide warning signs.

A sly disease

There are no urinary disorders in the beginning. Later, urinary problems may occur, identical to those with adenoma. In the advanced stages the pressure exercised by the ganglion metastases may result in edemas, phlebitis and bone metastases causing pain in the bones sometimes hard to control with painkillers.

Warning signs

The results of the digital rectal exam and PSA level may lead to performing a prostate biopsy, the only way for confirming or denying the disease. **Most often it is an adenocarcinoma.** The anatomy-pathology laboratory will also ascertain the degree of aggressiveness of the tumor.

In men who already have a benign tumor (adenoma), it is possible to discover cancer during a digital rectal exam; the doctor feels the adenoma, but also perceives

Better prevention: early screening

For socio-economic reasons, mass screening has not been introduced: systematic testing of all men after age 50 does not exist. The fact remains that early screening is based on personal initiative or because a doctor suggests it. Cancer prevention starts with an informative discussion letting the patient know screening is in his best interest.

a small hard lump. Another sign: the PSA level is not in proportion to the size of the adenoma. Lastly, an adenoma is systematically analyzed. Persistent **pain in the bones**, strong enough to wake a person up, is a sign of metastases. A digital rectal exam, PSA and prostate biopsy make it possible to know if there are metastases coming from the prostate.

Once a cancer diagnosis has been made, sometimes an intravenous urography, CAT scan, MRI, or bone scan *(see page 87)* needs to be performed to determine how far the cancer has spread. The treatment will not be the same if the cancer is localized in the prostate or if it has spread.

Fighting cancer

If the cancer appears to be completely localized in the prostate after all the tests, it is possible to cure it and various treatments are possible including surgery or radiation.

When the cancer has gone beyond the prostate, the treatments involve first slowing the advance of the disease (hormone treatment) and stopping pain.

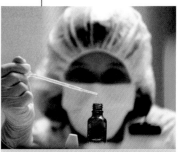

Monitoring cancer

Some cancers never advance, but it is difficult to know which ones will. Based on the patient's age, the number of biopsies performed, the Gleason score and digital rectal exam, sometimes it is preferable not to act, and a decision is made to simply monitor the patient (digital rectal exam + PSA test) without new biopsies being necessary.

This practice has been going on for many years in Scandinavian countries which has shown that certain prostate cancers actually do not advance.

Prostatitis

This is an infection of the prostate that has nothing to do with a benign tumor or cancer. It generally affects young men or those with a prostate adenoma.

There is no mistaking the signs

Acute prostatitis is due to a bacteria, either from the family of urinary tract bacteria (usually *Escherichia Coli*) or sexually transmitted bacteria.

Acute prostatitis starts like the flu, with muscle pain and a temperature, between 101° and 104°F. Next, signs of a urinary tract infection appear with burning sensations, frequent urge to urinate and urinating small amounts. Some men get up 10 to 15 times a night just to urinate a few drops.

A digital rectal exam reveals a sharp pain in the prostate showing an infection of the gland. A urine test needs to be performed to identify the bacteria in question, but they do not wait for the result before starting treatment. The physician generally prescribes a painkiller for the pain and an antibiotic which must be taken for at least three weeks. It is important to complete the treatment even if everything seems better after a few days, otherwise

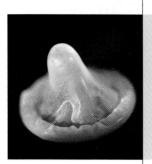

Precautionary measures for sexually transmitted germs

If the tests show that there are germs from a sexually transmitted disease, partners must also be treated even if they have no symptoms. If they are not treated they may later re-infect their partner. Sexual relations must be protected (by using condoms) for the entire length of the treatment.

a relapse is almost inevitable. The antibiotics need to fully penetrate the prostate and destroy the "hidden" germs. However, recurrence of the disorder, even several years later, is possible.

Chronic prostatitis

This may appear after repeated episodes of acute prostatitis but may also originate straightaway without really understanding what started it. A diagnosis is often difficult since the symptoms are vague: pain, sometimes limited to a simple nuisance or chronic heaviness in the sub-pubic region, perineal region or testes with intermittent pain or burning sensation. The prostate may be sensitive to the digital rectal exam and a sonogram may reveal prostatic calcifications. The tests (urine test, urethral sample and sperm culture) do not systematically reveal the presence of bacteria. Treatments involve long antibiotic therapies which are not always completely effective. Other treatments like hydrotherapy, acupuncture or even supplements (pollen or quercetin) are worth trying.

In some cases, the disorder is so bad that it literally ruins the life of afflicted men. Despite the drawbacks, some men decide to have their prostate totally removed.

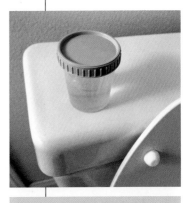

Abscesses

Prostate abscesses can develop during acute prostatitis. They are diagnosed by sonogram. Antibiotics may suffice to treat them but sometimes an endorectal puncture under sonogram or endoscopic removal is necessary to get rid of the abscess.

Increased PSA level

Around 5 to 10% of men in the United States suffer from prostatitis. It is important to point out that this prostate infection can also raise the PSA level. Sometimes it is impossible to determine the precise cause of the prostatitis.

Eat well for a healthy prostate

Certain foods eaten in quantity seem to actually protect men from prostate disorders.

The big winner: the tomato

This is the anti-prostatic food par excellence. Those who eat a lot of tomatoes, particularly tomato sauces, decrease their risk of prostate cancer. According to an American study of Health Professionals, men who consume tomato sauce and pizzas 2 to 4 times a week decrease their risk of prostate cancer by 35%. This beneficial effect of tomatoes is attributed to lycopene, a carotenoid pigment which is a powerful natural antioxidant. Lycopene also acts favorably on diagnosed cancer. Researchers gave 26 cancer patients 30 mg of lycopene per day and a placebo for a period of three weeks. First finding: the PSA level decreased in the group taking lycopene. All of these men were later operated on and the removed tumors were analyzed. Second finding: the tumors of the men who received the lycopene supplement showed signs of regression. A similar study was conducted using tomato sauce and the results were identical.

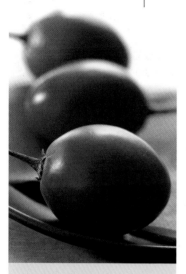

The tomato: better cooked

The lycopene in tomatoes is absorbed better by the body when the tomato is cooked and accompanied by a fat. Cooking actually releases the tomato pigments, and since lycopene is fat-soluble, fat helps with its absorption.

The benefits of a Chinese drink

Asia certainly appears to be a land filled with healthy foods! The antioxidant properties of green tea, the most popular drink in China, help give this country the lowest incidence of prostate cancer in the world.

The antioxidant substances, called catechins, in green tea stop the development of tumors. Studies conducted on mice with prostate cancer have shown that the equivalent of six cups of tea per day stopped the development of cancer cells. The treatment also made it possible to lengthen their lifespan compared to the other diseased mice.

Studies on men are still rare but daily intake of green tea may be an interesting means of prevention. And it is so easy to put into practice! So don't miss out, drink it!

More fish, less cancer

A Swiss study published in June 2001 in the prestigious medical journal *The Lancet* studied 6,272 men over 30 years. Those who regularly ate fatty fish (mackerel, sardines, tuna and salmon) had a 2 times lower risk of prostate cancer than those who ate little. The fats in these fish, fatty acids of the Omega 3 family, have anti-inflammatory and anti-tumor properties. Nuts, green vegetables and soybean oil and canola oil are equally rich in this substance.

More Omega 3 with flaxseeds

Thanks to their polyunsaturated fatty acids (Omega 3), flaxseeds lower testosterone blood levels. For an American pilot study (published in *Urology* in July 2001) 25 volunteers with cancer took 30 grams of flaxseed every day, a month before their operation, along with a low-fat diet. An analysis of their tumors showed a slowdown in cancer cell proliferation, as well as an increase in apoptosis (death of abnormal cells) compared to the other patients with the disease.

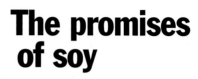

The promises of soy

Soy contains substances – isoflavones – which when ingested mimic estrogens. They are called plant estrogens. According to some studies these molecules may play a role in prostate health.

How did they come up with soy?

Epidemiology has shown that a Chinese man from Shanghai has a 10 times lower chance of developing prostate cancer than an American from San Francisco or Frenchman from Lille.

Researchers have tried to find what it is in the lifestyle of Asians that explains this advantage. They also observed that when Asians emigrate to the United States and adopt Western lifestyles, prostate cancer is 15 to 20 times more frequent than in their original country. And the data shows the same trend for benign prostatic hypertrophy.

Researchers deduced that this difference came from the diet of Asians, and in particular their high intake of **soy** which is a food rich in plant estrogens.

Soy: a noble food

The oldest Chinese pharmacoepia book, *Shen Nong Ben Cao*, mentioned soy around 2700 BC. Tofu has been made from soy for 4 thousand years and is the basis of the Chinese diet. It was introduced in Japan and Korea by Buddhist monks between the 2nd and 7th centuries. Tofu was recognized as a noble food in the court of the Chinese emperor.

In Asian countries soy has been the basis of the people's diet for many centuries: protein from soy accounts for 20 to 60% of total protein intake.

The benefits of isoflavones

For the past twenty years scientists have been actively examining soy and the benefits of isoflavones on health. Certain studies have led to the use of these molecules as a form of supplement since they are still used for women during menopause to combat hot flashes.

Things have not reached this point yet for the prostate, but the first research results look promising.

• A study showed *in vitro* that genistein, a soy isoflavone can slow the growth of cells taken from a hypertrophied prostate, as well as for prostate cancer cells. The higher the dose of the isoflavone in the culture the more the tissue growth is inhibited.

• In rats where prostate cancer was chemically induced, a genistein rich diet inhibited the development of cancer.

• For men, a study was conducted in 41 people with prostate cancer and with an increasing level of PSA. These men took 100 mg of soy isoflavones twice a day for 3 months. Researchers observed a slowdown in the progression of the PSA level.

Studies on men have just barely started. Clinical studies are in progress and it will be a few more years before researchers can clarify the potential role of soy in prostate diseases.

What is the Western intake of isoflavones?

It is estimated not to exceed 5 mg per day, while for Asian populations it is 25 to 45 mg per day. The Japanese have the highest intake of isoflavones with a daily consumption of soy by-products estimated at 200 mg per day.

Lastly, some authors believe that isoflavone consumption may even reach 250 mg per day for certain Asian populations.

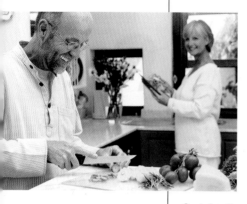

Natural prostate protectors

Certain vitamins and natural compounds have protective effects against cancer. In fruit, tea or supplements, these nutrients are healthy tricks that men should not go without.

Vitamin E

A certain number of studies have shown that vitamin E supplements, particularly in association with selenium, may play a protector role against prostate cancer. This vitamin fights free radicals which contribute to the onset of cancer. For a Finnish prevention study, (published in 1998 in *Journal of the National Cancer Institute*) 29,133 male smokers took 50 mg of vitamin E or a placebo on a daily basis for 6 years. The results showed that a daily intake of vitamin E made it possible to decrease the incidence of prostate cancer by 32% compared to the placebo group.

Zinc against cancer

Zinc, a mineral usually used to prevent wintertime complaints, showed an *in vitro* action on cancer proliferation mechanisms (study published in November 2002 in the journal *Clinical Cancer Research*). Like other antioxidants it can slow down the development of tumors.

Selenium

Selenium is a mineral found in soil and which we get from the fruits and vegetables we eat. Men with low selenium blood levels have a 4 to 5 times higher prostate cancer risk compared to the norm. Unfortunately, selenium blood levels decrease with age, and a supplement for older men may thus be a good idea.

A 1998 clinical study conducted by Dr. Larry Clark (University of Arizona Tucson) proved this point. A selenium supplement of 200 micrograms per day was administered and revealed that it is possible to reduce the risk of prostate cancer in men by 63%.

Vitamin D

This vitamin is mainly connected with calcium for its determinant role in healthy bones. The body synthesizes around 2/3 of the vitamin D it needs thanks to sunlight (as long as there is sufficient sunlight) and the rest from food. But it is also a strong weapon against cancer. Many American epidemiological studies have shown that people who live at higher latitudes are more likely to get cancer than those living closer to the equator. These people usually have a vitamin D deficiency due to the weaker sunlight. And this is definitely the case with prostate cancer: Florida is two times less affected than Maine, according to a study published in December 1992 in the journal *Cancer*.

The promises of quercetin

Quercetin is a substance synthesized by plants, which belongs to the large family of flavonoids. It possesses antioxidant properties. In 1999, a supplement based on quercetin, bromelain and papain (enzymes extracted from pineapple and papaya) was tested against a placebo on 30 patients with chronic prostatitis. 20% of the patients taking the placebo and 67% of those taking the supplement improved. However, this was a preliminary study.

Vitamin cocktail!

An American study (published in 1999 in *Cancer Epidemiology Biomarkers & Prevention*) showed that vitamin and mineral supplements have a protective effect against prostate cancer. Researchers compared the vitamin intakes of 697 men aged 40 to 64 with prostate cancer to 666 healthy men. The results showed that the regular intake of vitamins C and E and zinc is associated with a lower risk of prostate cancer.

Phytotherapy: Plants that help

Many plants have been demonstrated to be effective in the treatment of benign prostatic hypertrophy disorders. Some have been currently used for several years. A small guide to male phytotherapy.

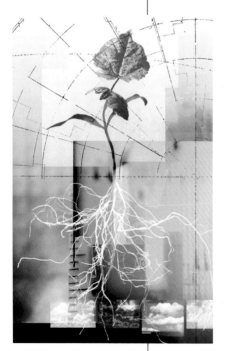

Saw palmetto *(Serenoa repens)*

Saw palmetto comes from the southeastern United States. Its small black berries have been used in traditional medicine to relieve irritations of the bladder, urethra and prostate. It is from the pulp and seeds of these ripe dried fruit that one of the main active ingredients is now extracted from the saw palmetto. It acts mainly on specific fatty acids by inhibiting the enzyme 5-alpha-reductase, making it possible to regulate the level of dihydrotestosterone in the prostate, the molecule responsible for increasing the volume of the prostate *(see page 30)*.

More than twenty clinical studies have shown that these extracts also make it possible to relieve urinary tract symptoms by reducing the contraction of the smooth muscles in the bladder and sphincter which cause urinary urgency.

Serenoa repens is part of the ingredients of classic medicines prescribed to treat prostate hypertrophy.

Pygeum *(Pygeum africanum)*

Pygeum africanum is a tree which grows in southern Africa, Madagascar and certain central African countries. Its bark is the active part. It contains compounds which act by inhibiting the growth factor in order to regulate prostate cell proliferation.

In September 2002, an overview of 18 clinical studies showed that pygeum extract, improved symptoms by 64% after 2 to 4 months of treatment (against only 30% in people taking the placebo). The urinary stream is sharply improved, with no side effects.

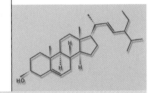

A common active ingredient: beta sitosterol

As its name indicates, beta sitosterol belongs to the family of phytosterols, compounds present in the cells of plants. They make it possible to maintain the structure of the cell membrane, just like cholesterol in humans.

Its action on the prostate is still not completely clear. However, it seems that beta sitosterol acts on certain prostate tissues or interferes with prostaglandins. These natural intermediates produced by the organism, act mainly in pain and inflammation phenomena at a gastric and gynecological level.

In 1999 a *British Journal of Urology* article reviewed 4 clinical studies where the results proved the effectiveness of beta sitosterol compared to a placebo for urinary disorders. The intensity of the disorders decreased. Researchers also observed an increase in urinary stream and a decrease in post-void residual. Beta sitosterol also helps to lower cholesterol.

More and more plants

Less exotic, they grow in our ditches and yards but have also turned out to be effective against prostatic hypertrophy.

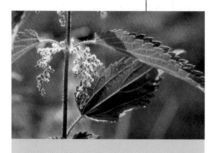

Nettle over the centuries

An essential food stuff for prehistoric humans, nettle was cultivated starting from the first centuries of the Christian era. The fibers of its stalk were used to weave cloth. Galen, a Greek doctor from the 2nd century AD reported its nutritional qualities. Later, its therapeutic properties became popular again, mainly to fight hemorrhages, headache, stomachache and even angina. Currently nettles can still be found on the table, in tarts or soups.

Nettle (*Urtica dioica*)

Here the root is used, the leaves are reserved for treating brittle nails and hair loss! Once again it is a sterol, beta sitosterol, which exercises its beneficial action on the prostate. A study which appeared in 1996 in the German journal *Urologue* showed that after 3 months of treatment with the nettle root, men observed their maximum urine stream increase by 66% (against only 36% in the placebo group). These effects, a decrease in prostate volume and improvement in urine stream, are comparable to those of the previous plants. A study appearing in 2000 in the *British Journal of Urology* compared the effects of a medicine (finasteride) with that of nettle extract and saw palmetto extract on 516 BPH patients. After 24 weeks, the patients of both groups observed an improvement in their condition in the same proportions, however, the plant extracts had the extra advantage in terms of side effects and tolerance.

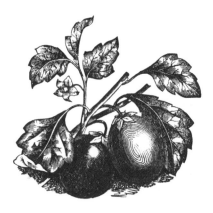

Pumpkin *(Cucurbita pepo)*

Brought from America, Native Americans ate its flesh and used its seeds to relieve kidney disorders. Later pumpkin seeds were used to get rid of intestinal worms. Currently, an oil with a high essential fatty acid content, is extracted from the seeds and used to improve prostate symptoms. Pumpkin seed oil has proven to be effective primarily in association with saw palmetto extract. Two studies, in 1989 and 1990, showed that after 3 months of treatment with pumpkin seed and saw palmetto extracts, the time and frequency of urination as well as urinary stream was sharply improved.

Plants: how to use them

All these plants are available in capsules which contain the complete powder or dry extracts. The complete powder is obtained through plant cryo-grinding (grinding at −321°F). This procedure makes it possible to obtain almost all the active ingredients. The dry extracts are obtained by vaporization or freeze drying. These methods make it possible to isolate and concentrate part of the active ingredients. Capsules should be taken at meals with some water.

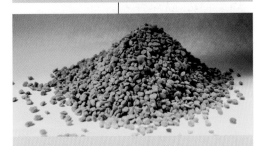

Pollen

Pollen extracts are now used as a current supplement, mainly to fight against fatigue and wintertime ailments. But pollen also acts on dihydrotestosterone receptors thus blocking hyperplasia. So, its effects are similar to the other two plants presented previously. According to a study published in 1996, in 86 men with BPH pollen led to a 78% improvement in urinary symptoms against a 55% improvement with pygeum extract. Pollen also stimulates the immune system and is an anti-oxidant.

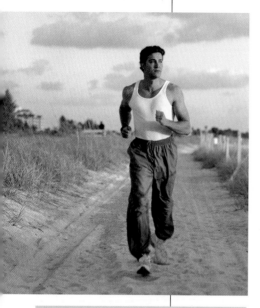

Daily health approaches

Urology literature at the beginning of the 20th century provided tips for a healthy lifestyle which are still valid today.

Drink lots, but stay away from alcohol!

• Avoid beverages such as white wine, beer, champagne and even pastis which contains a substance that slows down bladder activity, thus causing a risk of urine retention;

• Drink plenty: due to a fear of having to urinate, many men do not drink enough. The urine becomes very concentrated, which contributes to urinary tract infections. On the other hand you can stay away from soup at night which causes you to have to get up during the night...

Not too spicy

• Prevents constipation;

• Avoid spicy dishes: certain spices (like pepper), but also mustard contribute to burning sensations when urinating;

• Avoid long, full meals.

To stay in shape

Professor Edward Giovannucci (Harvard Medical School, Boston, Massachusetts), author of numerous studies on prostate and colon cancer summarized lifestyle measures that everyone should use in their daily life to stay healthy and prevent cancer in an article published in December 2002 *(The American Journal of Medicine)*:
- control your calorie intake and thus your weight;
- get regular exercise;
- cut down on your intake of red meat and cold cuts;
- eat more fruits and vegetables as well as whole grain cereals (instead of processed cereals).

And also think about...

• Practice a sport: the bladder is a muscle and physical activity makes it function better. Numerous studies have shown that men who get regular exercise suffer from fewer disorders related to prostatic hypertrophy. Walking is especially recommended: a study demonstrated that men who walk 2 to 3 hours a week have a 25% lower risk of getting BPH. Not to mention that this activity is also recommended to prevent cardiovascular risks. So start walking!

• Avoid sitting for long periods of time (long train or car trips) since this may cause acute urine retention;

• Avoid chills and the voluntary retention of urine;

• Also avoid vasoconstrictors, like those used for diarrhea and colds. They have an alpha stimulant activity (instead of an alpha blocker activity) and thus increase difficulty in urinating. So it is best to read the insert or box of all medicines before using them to make sure that they have no contraindication for prostate diseases. If the instructions for using the medicine warn against use by patients with prostate disease or disorder, talk to your physician about it.

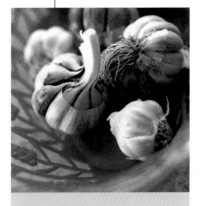

Spices and condiments with multiple virtues

Spices like pepper, paprika or Cayenne pepper can be irritants, however, do not neglect other plants that can spice up dishes. Garlic in particular like other plants of the amaryllis family (onions and shallots) have anti-cancer properties. A study published in 2002 in the *Journal of the National Cancer Institute* demonstrated that men who consume more than 10 g per day have a lower risk of developing prostate cancer. Beyond 10 g per day this risk decreases to 53% and lowers to 70% with the same quantity of onion!

Drugs for benign prostatic disease

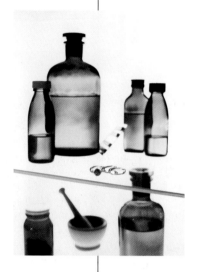

Two major families of drugs are used to relieve prostate disease. Alpha-blockers provide fast relief by relaxing the entire urinary tract. 5-alpha-reductase inhibitors act slowly, but directly, on the prostate.

A relaxed bladder

Initially used for high blood pressure, alpha-blockers, as their name indicates, act on alpha receptors in the arterial wall. By blocking their functioning, the drugs make it possible to lower blood pressure by dilatation of the arteries and less arteriole resistance. But they realized that alpha-blockers also improve urinary disorders in high blood pressure patients which a prostate adenoma. This led to the discovery that alpha receptors also exist in the prostate, neck of the bladder and bladder. These uro-genital receptors are slightly different than the ones in the arteries.

Blockage of the uro-genital receptors leads to a relaxation contributing to urine discharge. Urination starts better, the stream is stronger, the bladder empties better and post-void residual is less or even disappears. The action on the bladder receptors, lets the bladder be less "irritable", the frequency of nighttime urination decreases and control of the urge to urinate improves. There are various products on the market: Xatral®, Cardura®, Hytrin®, Flomax®.

Side effects which are more or less bothersome

They all have the same properties and identical side effects. The alpha-blocker effect can also be produced on the arteries thus creating low blood pressure phenomena characterized by malaise or dizziness, or less severe, by headache and a feeling of general fatigue. These side effects sometimes cause people to stop treatment. Another typical side effect is retrograde ejaculation, linked to blockage of the receptors of the bladder neck which closes poorly at the time of ejaculation. The sperm returns towards the bladder instead of being expelled towards the outside. These side effects are reversible when treatment is stopped.

When should one be treated?

Generally, if you don't have any urinary symptoms even if your prostate is enlarged, you will be left in peace.

If your symptoms are minor, they will certainly propose a plant based treatment or finasteride, and have your urologist monitor you.

If your daily life is greatly disturbed or the previous treatment did not work, they will prescribe alpha-blockers.

And surgery?

The decision to operate is not systematic. Your doctor will evaluate the social repercussions of your disorder, based on your activities. For example, the same treatment would not be proposed for a farmer who spends most of his time outdoors and an executive or teacher who would be obliged to leave the room various times in a morning to urinate. You can be certain they would be more likely to propose surgery in the latter case. Operations are always decided on a case by case basis.

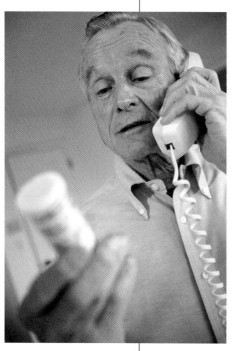

Reducing prostate volume

The second class of drugs: 5-alpha-reductase inhibitors. These drugs act differently: they are the only ones able to decrease the volume of the prostate.

5-alpha-reductase inhibitors

Finasteride (Proscar®) and dutaseride (Avodart®) have a radically different action than alpha-blockers. By reducing the dihydrotestosterone level inside the prostate, its volume is decreased. Even if, as we saw before, the volume of the prostate is not necessarily correlated to the intensity of the symptoms, reducing the volume of the prostate makes it possible to greatly improve urinary disorders. However, their action is slow, since at least 6 months to a year of treatment is needed to reduce the size of the prostate by 25%: a 50 gram prostate will become

Will finasteride prevent cancer?

A study is currently being conducted in the United States in order to evaluate the preventive role of finasteride (5-alpha-reductase inhibitor, used to treat prostate adenoma) on prostate cancer. The results will not be ready for a few years.

35 grams after several months. However these treatments rarely return the prostate to a normal size. They decrease the frequency of nighttime urination by improving the stream and reducing post-void residual.

The side effects are generally of a sexual nature with a decrease in the quantity of sperm and sometimes impotence, which can be reversed by stopping the treatment.

It is important to note that these drugs halve the PSA level. Thus some patients become alarmed when they see their PSA rise after stopping the treatment with finasteride or dutaseride. Actually, the PSA is just going back to its initial value.

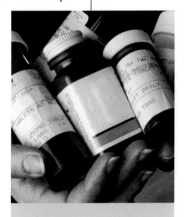

Finasteride and alpha-blocker association

This is used to combine the advantages of both drugs. Alpha-blockers act quickly (in a few days) and provide fast relief. Finasteride acts slowly "in-depth" on the prostate volume. There are natural medicines that can be taken for many years with no danger like saw palmetto or *Pygeum africanum*, two phytotherapy medicines also used to relieve prostate symptoms.

United we stand, divided we fall

In May 2002 the MTOPS (Medical Therapy of Prostatic Symptoms) study sponsored by the National Institutes of Health (NIH), showed that the treatment of BPH is more effective if alpha-blocker drugs are combined with finasteride. 3,047 men over age 50 with BPH took the treatment for 4 1/2 years. The results showed that compared to a placebo, the alpha-blocker drug reduced the risk of clinical BPH progression by 39%, finasteride by 34% and combined treatment by 67%.

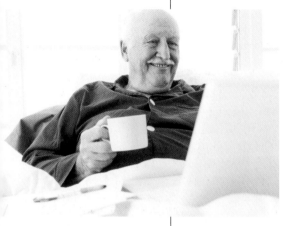

Relieving acute urinary retention

Acute urinary retention is a direct consequence of benign prostatic hypertrophy. It is very painful and requires prompt intervention.

The catheter

This is the only way to relieve the pain caused by acute urinary retention. Sometimes your physician can insert the catheter, otherwise you need to go to the emergency room. Catheterization, if the catheter is inserted with no problems, is not painful and more importantly it brings such relief that some patients want to go home, thinking that the problem is "solved". But the bladder is very bloated and weak due to this ordeal. If the catheter is removed, the retention will reoccur as soon as the bladder is full again. Thus the catheter is left in for a few days to let the bladder heal. It is removed after urination becomes normal again.

However, this does not mean that the initial cause has been solved by any means, and the hypertrophied prostate may cause urine retention again at any time. If normal urination

After catheterization: blood in the urine bag

When the bladder is very bloated and when it is continuously emptied, small veins in the bladder mucous membrane can "break" and result in major hematurias with clots. To prevent this phenomenon, the bladder is emptied only in stages: the flow must be stopped every 100 to 200 ml and for a few minutes each time.

does not start when the catheter is removed, it needs to be reinserted and the BPH operated on.

When it is not possible to operate: a permanent catheter

For patients who do not start normal urination after the catheter is removed and whose general conditions do not allow surgery, the catheter can be left in permanently. In this case it needs to be changed every month and sometimes a weak dose antibiotic treatment is prescribed as a preventive measure.

Self-catheterization

Some non-operable patients, or those who do not want surgery, can learn to catheterize themselves with the initial help of a doctor. An average of 4 to 6 catheterizations are required per day.

A permanent catheter in practice

A risk of infection exists, but it is decreased by changing the catheter each month, regular washing of the tip of the penis and sometimes taking antibiotics in small doses as a preventive measure. A permanent catheter does not hinder everyday activities. During the day it is connected to a "day bag" attached to the calf and is emptied by a small tap on the bottom part. During the night, the bag is replaced with a "night bag", with a greater capacity, so that it is not necessary to get up to empty it.

And if the catheter cannot be inserted?

In some cases a catheter cannot be inserted due to internal anatomical reasons. In this case a sub-pubic catheter is used. After locally anesthetizing the sub-pubic region, a trocar (sharp-pointed surgical instrument) is inserted above the pubis which penetrates the bladder and a drain is placed to empty the urine.

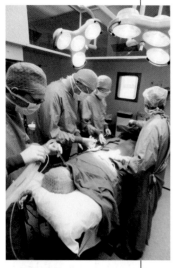

When surgery is required

Adenoma surgery only involves the adenoma and not the entire prostate.

When should one be operated on?

• In the case of acute retention, when normal urination is not resumed after removal of the catheter.

• If the urinary symptoms have too strong an impact on everyday life, if they are not improved by drugs or get worse despite treatment.

• In the case of repeated urinary tract infections, bladder stones, repeated hematurias, chronic retention or kidney failure.

Selecting an operating technique

This choice depends on the volume of the prostate and the practices of the surgeon. Briefly, BPH with a small and average volume are operated on "through natural orifices" (endoscopic reduction) and large BPH are operated on by opening the abdomen (the limit is around 60 grams).

Adenoma reduction

This is an operation through a natural orifice. The operation is performed using an endoscopy with a resectioner – metallic tube equipped with an optical system and cutting electrode at the tip. It is used to reduce the interior of the prostate. It is called endoscopic resection. For safety reasons, it cannot last more than an hour, this is why it is not indicated for large adenomas, which

Consultation with the anesthesiologist

This is mandatory before any operation.
Be sure the anesthesiologist sees all of your records before any operation. The doctor will ask you if you have had previous operations, if you are allergic to certain substances and about any drugs you are currently taking. This will be the basis for deciding the type of anesthesia: general or local.

require a much longer and thus dangerous resection.

The anesthetized patient is put in gynecological position and the resectioner is inserted in the urethra. First the interior of the bladder is checked, then the two lobes of the prostate are resected which can be seen very clearly projecting in the urethra. These lobes are cut up into small shavings which are pushed into the bladder. They are removed at the end of the operation using a special syringe before being sent to the laboratory for analysis. Most patients are dismissed from the hospital a few days after the operation, or even a little later if the urine continues to remain red for too long.

Removal of large adenomas

This operation requires a small horizontal or vertical opening of a few centimeters above the pubis. It is generally performed under general anesthesia. The tumor is removed in one piece in order to be analyzed. Due to the incision, the hospitalization is a little longer. Surgical removal of an adenoma is quick and may take 15 to 30 minutes.

An adenoma is systematically analyzed

The removed adenoma is sent to the anatomy-pathology laboratory to be analyzed. In some cases, a small quantity of cancer cells is found by chance. Based on the case, your urologist will decide to simply monitor you or to prescribe new tests. A decision for a new operation may be made to remove the rest of the prostate.

The treatment of stones

This is done at the same time as the treatment for the adenoma which caused them.

- During a resection, a lithotrite (an instrument with an ultrasound system) is inserted through a natural orifice and crushes the stones when it comes into contact with them in the bladder. The small pieces are removed in the same way as the shavings.

- They are simple to remove surgically when the bladder is opened.

The alternatives to BPH surgery

BPH operations are not suggested for young patients. Operating techniques such as transurethral incision or thermotherapy are preferred.

Transurethral incision

This is used on small adenomas and makes it possible to maintain normal ejaculation in more than 80% of patients. It is a technique using the natural orifice where the adenoma is not reduced. A "trench is dug" at the cervix of the adenoma. This trench provides a better opening for urine and improves the blocking symptoms. It is limited to small adenomas. It is ineffective on larger ones. The hospital stay is brief.

Prostate stent

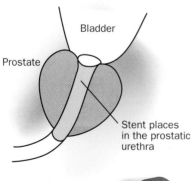

Bladder

Prostate

Stent places in the prostatic urethra

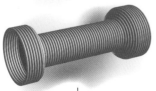

Stents

These are placed at the level of the prostatic urethra using an endoscope and keep the lobes of the prostate separated, thus decreasing the obstruction.

They can be placed under general, epidural or local anesthesia. It is a simple operation and the patient can leave the next day.

They are used with men who are too "weak" for the traditional operations.

However, this simple operation has frequent complications:

• migration of the stent in the bladder (mainly for large adenomas), requiring its removal by endoscopy;

• repeated urinary tract infections, due to the presence of a foreign body;

• stone build-up on the stent for the same reason;

• growth of tissue through the stent mesh, which may cause an obstruction and then require endoscopic resection.

These complications make it difficult to consider as a permanent or even long-term treatment.

And laser?

Laser, delivered at a temperature of around 570°F, causes tissue destruction similar to that obtained with surgery. There is less bleeding and the hospital stay is shorter. This technique is not used much due to the high cost of the material. Like the previous technique it has the drawback of not taking out the tissue (because it is destroyed by heat) and thus it is not possible to anatomically and pathologically analyze it.

Microwave thermotherapy

Using heat, it is possible to obtain a necrosis (destruction) of the tissue. The early machines heated to 115°F but the results were not conclusive. Thus it became necessary to heat to 160-175°F to effectively destroy the tissues. Cooling systems are required to protect the neighboring structures like the urethra and rectum. Anesthesia is necessary. The overall results of this technique are not as good as surgery, but it can be proposed to replace treatment with drugs (thus avoiding the need to take medicine regularly) or for a patient who does not want to undergo surgery. The rate of retrograde ejaculation ranges from 0 to 45% and post-op retention is possible which requires wearing a sub-pubic catheter for several days.

Treatments for localized prostate cancer

The goal is to eradicate the disease in order to obtain full recovery: 2 possibilities: surgical removal or the "destruction" of the gland by radiation.

The prostate cancer operation

Unlike benign hypertrophy, prostate cancer surgery involves removal of the entire gland and seminal vesicles. It is called a total prostatectomy.

Based on the practices and experience of the surgeon, it is performed:
- "open" with an incision from the pubis to the navel;
- by going through the perineum;
- using a celoscope, many small incisions are made in the abdomen wall to insert instruments. The operation is performed under a camera lens. The surgeon watches his work on a television screen.

The hospital stay lasts a few days for operations through the perineum and with celoscope and about a week for open abdominal surgery.

A month after the operation the PSA should have dropped to 0.

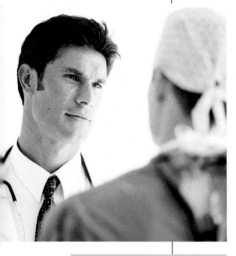

A clear choice

Cancer treatment must be selected together with your physician, the urologist and your partner. The physician must clearly explain the advantages, drawbacks and risks of each therapeutic solution so that the patient makes an informed choice he does not later regret.

Radiation therapy

This is an alternative to surgery, with long term results and similar recovery rate. It involves destroying the cancer cells using high energy rays. The treatment lasts around 6 weeks, so that the radiation is administered to the patient in small quantities each day to minimize complications. The complications are basically cystitis (bladder inflammation) or proctitis (rectum inflammation), normally temporary, but which can be disabling in exceptional cases. It is difficult to predict repercussions on sexuality, since the rays act slowly over several months. However, the risk of impotence does exist.

Unlike surgery, the PSA lowers much more slowly, even over an entire year.

Surgery or radiation?

This depends on the patient's life expectancy and his own choice. The longer the life expectancy the more the urologist tends to operate, saving the radiation option for taking care of any recurrences in later years. However, the risk of impotence frightens some men who then choose radiation.

Starting at age 70 radiation is suggested more often since the operation-related risks increase and the life expectancy is shorter, but some men in good health are operated at that age.

Around age 80, men may choose not to undergo surgery and to be monitored regularly, since the disease evolves very slowly at that age. Radiation or hormone treatment (*see page 70*) may also be suggested.

Other techniques

These are currently being studied. This involves Brachytherapy, a technique which uses ultrasound that kills the tissues by heating them and radium therapy. This is done under anesthesia and with ultrasonic control by implanting radioactive iodine seeds in the prostate which deliver localized radioactivity to the gland and thus reduce the risk of rectum and bladder burns in external radiation therapy. This technique has the advantage of maintaining erectile functioning in 70% of cases. Its effectiveness on long-term cancer needs to be evaluated.

Continue monitoring

Once the cancer is treated, it is imperative to continue to be monitored and to have a regular digital rectal exam and PSA test in order to detect any relapse.

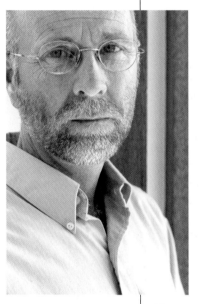

Treatment of advanced cancer

At this stage of cancer, recovery is no longer possible. It is only possible to stop its advance.

Hormone, or rather anti-hormone treatment

Prostate cancer is complexly tied to hormone secretions. Thus the treatments involve suppressing hormone production by using adapted drugs. They do not cure the cancer but only block it for a period that can range from several months to numerous years. The duration of the action depends on the aggressiveness of the tumor and its sensitivity to the medicines.

These treatments are used in locally developed forms or with metastases, i.e. the forms where the cancer has gone past the local area and can no longer be expected to be cured. It is also given to certain patients with less developed cancer, in an operation or radiation preparation phase.

At the beginning of the 20th century cancer was treated by surgical castration. Later, up until 20 years ago, urologists removed the testicular pulp, the tissue that produces testosterone. It was a less psychologically traumatizing operation than castration. Currently, the drugs used basically create a "chemical" castration. They also cause a drop in testicular volume as well as other secondary effects of castration: hot flashes, weight gain, increase in fat at the thighs and hips and loss of hairiness.

Two main families of drugs

LHRH *(Luteinizing Hormone Releasing Hormone)* is a hormone responsible for controlling other hormones, particularly LH *(Luteinizing Hormone)* which initiates the synthesis of testosterone.

The first class of drugs: the **"LHRH analogues"** These products attach to the pituitary gland to take the place of real LHRH. They completely halt the production of LH, which cause the testicles to decrease in size and stop the production of testosterone. So the cancer cells become "dormant".
LHRH analogues are administered by injection every month or every three months.

Second class: **antiandrogens.** These molecules attach to all the androgen receptors of the organ, including those of the prostate. The male hormones can no longer exercise their action because their place has been "taken" by the drug. Since the cancer cells are no longer stimulated by the body's androgens, they become dormant.

Combined treatment

LHRH analogues and antiandrogens can be given together or separately. Generally, these treatments should not be stopped, except in special cases where they can be given intermittently. Sometimes they can be given as preparation for surgery or together with radiation therapy. In this case they are used with a neoadjuvant goal.

Other solutions

Estrogens, drugs composed of synthetic estrogens, cortisone, products used to increase skeletal calcification and chemotherapy are only used in resistant advanced forms or those which are no longer hormone sensitive.

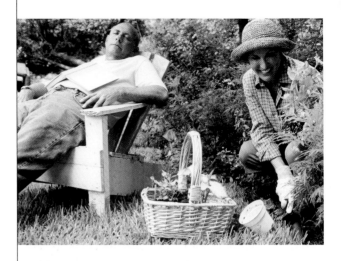

Post-op complications

What are the consequences of an adenoma operation or total removal of the prostate when it is cancerous on the urinary system and sexuality?

Male fertility decreases with age

Scientific studies on the subject are unanimous: a man is not as fertile at 80 as he was at 20. The overall quality of sperm decreases over the years: there are fewer spermatozoids and they are not as mobile. The probability of having sperm motility problems reaches 80% at age 50 and practically 100% at age 80. There are many factors which jeopardize fertility.

After an adenoma operation: often sterile, rarely impotent

The operation for prostatic hypertrophy does not cause impotence and does not hinder sexual relations. However, medicine is not an exact science, and a very low percentage of patients become impotent without being able to explain why. Retrograde ejaculation is a basic complication of adenoma surgery: the sperm go into the bladder instead of being ejaculated. This does not alter the quality of the sexual relation, but it does make the man sterile. This is why doctors try to avoid operating on young patients who may still want to have children.

Around 20% of patients operated by transurethral incision become sterile.

No more prostate, no more erection

Total removal of the prostate causes impotence problems in 80% of cases. The operation often damages the nerves that control erectile function, to a varying degree based on the technique used. Saving a nerve is sometimes possible, but not without risk since the cancer cells may remain in the nerve that has been saved. Moreover, it is difficult to achieve this since the nerves are very thin and the bleeding caused by the surgery makes it hard to see them.

Prostate removal requires tying the vas deferens, thus causing infertility. However, some patients do have erections after and a sexual life. If they sometimes observe an ejaculation, this is due to the fact that the periurethral gland also produces part of the components of sperm. However, this ejaculate does not contain any spermatozoids.

Complications related to the surgery and anesthesia

Complications which are common to all operations and anesthesia are increasingly rare. The most important risks are phlebitis and pulmonary embolism, requiring systematic post-op anticoagulant treatment. In order to prevent hemorrhage-related complications, the patient is closely monitored and can be given a transfusion if needed.

Urinary incontinence

Urinary incontinence, the greatest worry that makes patients fear the operation is rare, since it occurs after only 0.5 to 1% of adenoma operations and in less than 3% after total prostate removal for cancer.

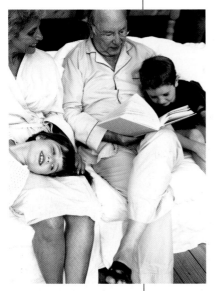

Rediscovering a normal life

After a prostate operation the three key words are prevent, rehabilitate and monitor.

Preventing urinary tract infections

Urinary tract infections are particularly frequent after a prostate operation, mainly because the microbial flora is more significant in a bladder that empties poorly. The introduction of an instrument into the urethra and a catheter on the days after the operation "wakes up" the bacteria again. This is why recovering patients are almost systematically given a preventive antibiotic treatment. A urine test is done when the catheter is removed, since hygiene measures do not eliminate all the risks of infections. Thus certain patients leave the hospital with an antibiotic treatment to take at home.

Since urinary tract infections are common and closely linked with this type of operation, you should not jump to conclusions and call it a "hospital infection". The infections may involve the testicle (orchitis) or epididymis (epididymitis) and turn into a significant testicular pain. They are treated with antibiotics and anti-inflammatory drugs.

Starting to urinate again

After leaving the clinic or hospital you must wait from 1 to 3 months before you can urinate normally again. You must avoid all physical strain after the operation to prevent the operated area from bleeding, which takes a long time to form a scar.

During this period urine tests will reveal any pus, but this is not a sign for worry.

You will have to learn to hold your urine again, with "stop-urinate" exercises. When urinating you stop the stream by tightening the sphincters, then you release them, then you stop again, etc. You can start these exercises at your home before the operation to make post-op rehabilitation easier. In the event of dripping, more intensive rehabilitation may be prescribed with a specialized therapist.

Sexual activity can be resumed after around a month, but ejaculation will be retrograde.

A yearly check-up

It is rare for the adenoma to grow back, but it is possible over several years. Annual monitoring will continue to be necessary. Your prostate has not been totally removed. Only the adenoma is taken out. The egg has been removed, but the shell remains: it is possible to develop cancer in this peripheral prostatic shell. Thus you need to continue to see your urologist who will perform a digital rectal exam and test your PSA once a year.

So, you ask, why didn't you just take everything out? Total removal of the prostate is only justified in the case of cancer. The sexual and psychological repercussions are usually overwhelming. So it is better to avoid this whenever possible.

Narrowing of the urethras

With time stenoses of the urethra or hardening of the opening (scarring on the neck of the bladder) may occur. These are fiber reactions which obstruct the discharge of urine. Just like a scar on the skin may sometimes result in an unaesthetic growth, here this growth is in the urethral canal and its consequence is obstruction. This narrowing which causes urinary disorders is diagnosed with a cystoscopy. They can be treated by endoscopy (through natural orifices) under anesthesia with a few days of hospitalization.

After cancer, a check-up every 6 months

One month after the operation, the PSA needs to have lowered to 0. It will continue to be monitored every six months along with a digital rectal exam to check for relapse. Radiation or hormonal treatment will be prescribed if necessary.

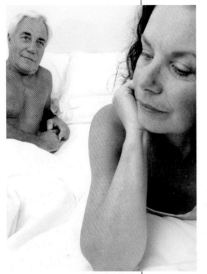

When sexuality is affected

Prostate disorders in a fifty-year old are not symptoms of impotence. The causes may be multiple.

Get rid of old ideas

Operations on prostate adenomas do not make men impotent and they can continue a normal sexual life. The only repercussion may be retrograde ejaculation: the sperm is no longer ejaculated to the outside but sent to the bladder. This phenomenon has no important physical consequences, but certainly means sterility.

Now it is true that in the age ranges affected by prostate diseases, erection disorders are frequent, but there are multiple reasons:
- various psychological factors (retirement, problems with life, etc.);
- a decrease in desire within the couple;
- the impact of certain diseases like diabetes or certain addictions such as smoking or alcoholism.

The urinary disorders caused by BPH often do not help things. The irritation due to frequent getting up at night which disturbs the sleep of both partners may result in a certain negative reaction towards the uro-genital system and in turn affect sexuality.

In addition, this may explain why some patients who had sexual problems, rediscover a normal sexual activity after having their adenoma operation.

Sexuality after prostate cancer

Men who have had cancer become impotent in 80% of cases after complete removal of the prostate. The erector nerves, which are very thin and sit against the prostate are often damaged during the operation. Certain techniques may save them, but this is rare. After radiation treatment 30 to 60% become impotent and 100% after hormone treatment.

The first enemy for erection: stress

Total impotence is rare and is manifested by a complete absence of erection, during sexual relations, or during the night and in the early hours. More often, erection disorders are characterized by an "erectile insufficiency", which means an erection which starts but does not continue. The tumescence phase is normal, hardness barely starts but "falls" at the time of penetration. The cause is usually psychological. Stress (even if unconscious) and fear of failure cause certain substances to be released in the blood which have a negative role on the rigidity of the cavernous body. The more the man finds himself in a failure situation the worse the phenomenon gets.

Two therapies can be used at the same time: sex therapy and drugs designed to help or cause erections.

How does a normal erection occur?

Normally erections occur during sexual relations, following physical and psychological stimulations. Outside of sexual relations, erections also occur naturally at night during sleep and in the morning when waking up. Erection is when rigidity of the penis is obtained making penetration during sex possible.

The penis is composed of two hollow bodies, real sponges which are filled with blood during sexual stimulation. They increase in volume (tumescence), then become rigid (rigidity) which makes penetration and keeping the erection possible. After ejaculation, the phenomena reverse: the blood leaves the hollow bodies which become softer (detumescence) until returning to the rest state (flaccidity).

The ejaculation mechanism

Ejaculation is the emission of sperm through the urethral opening. The sperm is discharged thanks to a spasm of the muscle in the perineum region and canals in which it is found. Upstream, the smooth sphincter of the neck of the bladder is closed. Forcing the sperm to be driven to the exterior.

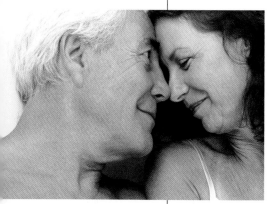

Against erection breakdowns

Impotence is not a fatality. Psychological therapy and drugs complement each other to restore confidence to the two partners and get to the bottom of the problem.

How do you get things back on an even keel?

• Drugs like sildenafil (Viagra®) may provide good results. Complying with the cardiovascular contraindications is imperative and never use the product without talking to your physician about it beforehand. After a total prostatectomy, it is effective in 50% of cases as long as the highest dosage form is taken.

• Inter-cavernous injections of prostaglandins or alpha-blockers have good results. The product is injected into the penis and starts dilation of the cavernous body, where blood flows in causing an erection. Not painful (except in exceptional cases), they are not always well-accepted, since the fact of having to "shoot up" in the penis 10 minutes before sex makes the act slightly less romantic.

Sex therapy

Sex therapy tries to analyze how the problem started: fighting within the couple, work conditions driving apart the two partners and resulting in command sex and psychological problems (emotional shock or problems at work). A sex therapy doctor then tries to learn how the problem is perpetuated: how the man reacts to the problem, his partner, the ability to talk about it and efforts made by one or the other to improve their sexual and affective relationship. In brief, they need to relearn how to be a couple!

Besides, it is no longer the woman who is causing the erection, but the needle. Thus the erection is no longer considered as a natural phenomenon, but as something artificial, which leads many couples to abandon this.

Viagra and friends: without stimulation, no action

Stimulation during foreplay releases certain substances, and without these substances Viagra cannot become effective. This underlines the importance of starting the act in order for the drug to act, and is why sildenafil, like apomorphine chlorohydrate are considered as erection "helpers". These drugs must be taken one hour before having sex and will only work if there is sexual stimulation. Even though Viagra is very famous it is not the only 5-phosphodiesterase inhibitor: tadalafil (Cialis®) and vardenafil (Levitra®) are also used to help erections.

Prostheses

A penile prosthesis is a surgical solution that involves implanting inflatable supports in the cavernous body. They are filled by a small pump placed between the testicles. The use of these prostheses has become rarer since the introduction of inter-cavernous body injections.

The magic pellet

On the more serious side, this is the intrauretral injection of prostaglandin gel (MUSE). The pellet is the size of a large grain of rice which is inserted with an applicator, into the urethra, about half an hour before sex. It is composed of a prostaglandin gel (like the intra-cavernous injections). This gel spreads slowly through the urethra wall and reaches the cavernous body. It is not quite as effective as the injections, but is better accepted psychologically.

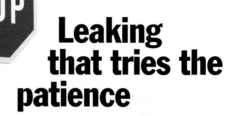

Leaking that tries the patience

Urinary incontinence is defined as the inability to retain urine. Unlike popular notions, it is rare. If it happens to you, don't be embarrassed and do not hesitate to talk about it because there are solutions.

Incontinence after an operation is rare

This fear, if it exists, is evidentially based on experienced, heard or recounted examples, but it is necessary to put things into perspective. The risk of incontinence after adenoma surgery is low: 0.5 to 1%. It increases with the age of the operated person, since the striated sphincter of the urethra has less force in a 90 year old man than in a 65 year old.

The risk after a cancer operation (total prostatectomy) is less than 3%. Small leaks of a few drips at the end of the day requiring the use of absorbent pads are more frequent (10 to 20%) but they do not impact the comfort of daily life.

For younger men

Younger men may try an artificial sphincter. It is not a major operation and its greatest risk is infection, just like for all prostheses. This operation involves going through the perineum and fitting a small silicon sleeve around the urethra, used to control opening and closing with a small pump around one centimeter in diameter located between the testicles.

The solutions

The "stop-urinating" method discussed earlier is often sufficient. The ideal is to start practicing before the operation, and definitely to continue afterwards.

If this is not enough you will need around fifteen perineum and sphincter rehabilitation sessions with a physical therapist specialized in the field who possesses the necessary material. Do not expect the physical therapist to come to your house since the material is in his or her office and you will have to go there. This rehabilitation is usually very effective.

In some very exceptional cases, it will still not be sufficient. In older men, it is possible to just use absorbent pads, or condom catheters if the number of pads used per day is too high. But the condom catheters do not always hold well, so a permanent catheter may be required, which needs to be changed regularly to avoid the risk of infection. This catheter is connected to a plastic bag attached to your calf during the day, which allows greater autonomy and a completely normal life.

On the subject of rehabilitation

If rehabilitation is started before the operation (5 to 6 sessions), the results on post-op continence will be better. The results tend to deteriorate over time and maintenance sessions may be necessary every year. If the rehabilitation is not effective within 30 sessions, it will continue to be so, thus it is useless to continue it.

Specialized stores

Pads can be found in drugstores and supermarkets. It is important to note that there are specialized stores in big cities where they can show you complete product ranges suited for male anatomy and give you the clearest advice based on your specific incontinence.

THE PROSTATE:
ANSWERS TO YOUR QUESTIONS

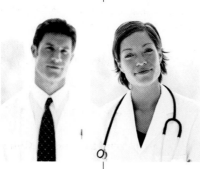

Why do they need to examine my prostate when my blood test was normal?

A normal PSA does not keep you from having benign prostatic hypertrophy or prostate cancer.

Is it dangerous to have PSA?

PSA is not toxic for the body. It reflects the condition of the prostate. If it is high a prostate exam is warranted, but if this exam is okay, you won't need a drug to "treat this PSA". It just needs to be monitored.

My prostate is enlarged. Why don't you give me some medicine?

A benign prostatic hypertrophy without a urinary disorder does not need treatment.

I am taking a prostate drug, one of these days I'll need an operation, wouldn't it be better to do it now?

All BPH do not necessarily become complicated nor is surgery mandatory. BPH are only operated on if they cause urine retention, repeated infection or BPH with urinary symptoms which respond increasingly poorly to drugs.

Since my operation I am no longer a man. You told me I would no longer have erections, but you never told me I wouldn't get a hard-on!!!

This real comment, shows not only that a discussion before the operation is important, but that it is also necessary to make sure the terms used are understood. Some people mix up erection and ejaculation!

You found a prostate cancer, yet nothing is bothering me. It seems like they make good drugs now that work well!

Prostate cancer drugs are only used for advanced forms where an operation is not reasonable since recovery is no longer possible.

If you feel fine, that is rather reassuring and if the cancer test is normal, only total removal of the prostate will cure this disease that is not yet bothering you in the least. Your long term life expectancy depends on it.

I don't understand, I was opened up and my friend, he was operated by the canal!

Your friend had an endoscopic resection because he had a small or medium size adenoma. You had to be "opened up" because your adenoma was too big to be operated on by endoscopy or because your prostate was cancerous and it was necessary to perform a total prostatectomy.

If the prostate doesn't work anymore can it be treated with laser?

The techniques using laser are not currently practiced and are only used in certain cases. The reference operations for the prostate are:
• for benign hypertrophy: endoscopic resection and surgical adenomectomy;
• for cancer: total prostatectomy.

I was operated on, but can my prostate grow back?

Regrowth is possible, but rare, after BPH surgery. If urinary disorders reoccur, it is most likely due to stenosis of the urethra or hardening of the opening.

I was operated on for an adenoma, and I had to return to have everything taken out. Why didn't you just do it all at once?

You were actually operated on for an adenoma and your prostate showed no signs of cancer, so a total removal was not justified. Systematic analysis of adenomas sometimes makes it possible to discover small cancerous foci that no other exam would have been able to detect. Consider yourself lucky to have discovered cancer in the early stage when you can still be cured, but certainly, at the inconvenience and risk of another operation.

I have cancer which they decided not to operate on, will I have to have more biopsies?

No, more biopsies won't be necessary, the only check-up exams you'll need are a digital rectal exam and PSA test.

Can the prostate cause incontinence all by itself?

Prostate disease incontinences are caused by urinary urgencies, which are impossible to battle for a long time: the pressure from the bladder contraction can be so strong that you'll have to find a bathroom as soon as possible. These urgencies often react well to alpha-blocker drugs.

The phenomena of dripping a few drops after urinating or later are not defined as incontinence.

Urinary incontinence is an overflow of urine discharged due to a constantly filled bladder (chronic retention). Drug or surgical treatments can be used to solve the problem of incontinence as the consequence of prostate disease.

Will my sexual problems get better after the operation?

No, sexual problems are not related to the prostate. The aim of the operation is only to relieve the urinary disorders and not sexual problems which are often psychological.

I have chronic prostatitis, can you give me some healthy lifestyle tips?

Like all prostate disorders, you need to avoid spicy foods, white wine and champagne as well as sports such as cycling and horseback rising. Sex is not contraindicated, but you may need to use condoms in the acute phase.

Does having prostatitis increase the risk of getting an adenoma?

A prostatitis does not increase the risk of getting an adenoma or cancer. On the other hand, the prostate needs to be monitored, since the consistency of the gland, in chronic prostatitis, can be firm and PSA can increase as it does when cancerous. Thus chronic prostatitis can mask cancer, so regular monitoring is important.

GLOSSARY
OF MEDICAL TESTS
IN UROLOGY

URODYNAMIC TEST

Why?

To predict the possible effectiveness of an operation on the prostate if its responsibility in urinary disorders is not clear.

To evaluate the condition of the sphincter in post-op incontinence.

How?

It is a complex, painless test that involves placing a small catheter in the bladder through the urethra. This catheter is used to record the pressures prevailing in the urethra and bladder during bladder filling and urination.

URINARY OUTPUT

Why?

To study the urinary output, i.e. the volume urinated in relation to unit of time. This test makes it possible to identify a dysuria, where the characteristics and significance are not always easy to obtain through questions.

How?

This is a simple test performed at the urologist's office which consists of urinating into a funnel connected to an instrument which traces a curve.

CYSTOSCOPY

Why?

A cystoscopy reveals:

• the appearance of a trabeculated bladder;

• bladder stones;

• significant projection of the prostate in the urethra;

• narrowing of the urethra responsible for dysuria; for this indication it is increasingly replacing the retrograde urography;

• a bladder tumor causing a hematuria.

A cystoscopy must be systematic for all hematurias before saying it is caused by the prostate.

How?

This involves inserting a cytoscope (a flexible optical fiber instrument) into the urethra used to evaluate the extension of the prostatic hypertrophy and the interior of the bladder. It is performed under local anesthesia of the urethra using xylocaine gel, lasts a few minutes and is done in the doctor's office.

INTRAVENOUS UROGRAPHY (IVU)

Why?

This is an x-ray of the entire urinary tract, from the kidneys to the bladder and urethra. This examination is used to view all the "canals" but it does not include any image of the prostate (only images of pushing back around the prostate are visible). It is very useful for understanding the impact of a prostatic hypertrophy on the urinary tract canals and ducts and on bladder functioning.

The intravenous urography makes it possible to look for:

• bladder stones;

• post-urination residual;

• bloating of the ureters, renal pelvises and calices;

• delayed functioning of the kidneys in advanced cases;

• pushing back of the bladder floor or lifting of the ureter ends due to a enlarged prostate;

• existence of another pathology which could have the same symptoms as prostatic hypertrophy.

How?

This is performed at the radiologist's. You need to have fasted. A creatinine test needs to be done beforehand and sometimes an allergy drug is prescribed. Iodine allergies must be reported when the appointment is made. The test lasts around 20 minutes and is performed with an iodine IV. This product circulates in the blood and after a few minutes is eliminated in the kidneys into the urinary tract.

It is used to view the kidneys and their canals or ducts (calices, renal pelvises and ureters). X-rays of the kidneys, ureters, bladder and urethra are taken before, during and after urination.

RETROGRADE UROGRAPHY

Why?

This is only required in a few special cases. It is performed to look for urethra narrowing which may cause a dysuria identical to that of prostatic hyper-trophy.

How?

The radiologist puts a catheter into the urinary open-ing and injects an iodine product used to view the urethra and bladder.

CAT SCAN AND MAGNETIC RESONANCE IMAGING (MRI)

Why?

These more complex exams are usually required for a prostate cancer test. These two medical imaging techniques give a more precise idea of the contents of the abdomen and pelvis and may help in selecting a surgical treatment, radiation therapy or the use of certain drugs. The CAT scan is not very helpful for examining the prostate but it is useful for understanding its environment. MRI is more informative in terms of the prostate and an endorectal MRI can provide additional valuable information.

How?

The patient must fast before the CAT scan and an injection of an iodine product is necessary. For the MRI, patients must report any metallic objects they have in their bodies (pacemakers, prostheses, etc.).

BONE SCAN

Why?

To screen for prostate cancer bone metastases.

How?

This painless examination involves obtaining an image of the entire skeleton on a single x-ray. A weak dose of radioactive product is injected intravenously, with no danger for the patient or his family.

PROSTATE BIOPSY

Why?

A biopsy is performed to diagnose prostate cancer.

How?

This involves taking samples of the prostate with a fine needle. It is done endorectally with a sonogram used to guide the operation in very precise areas of the prostate. 6 to 8 samples are taken at the same time. Anesthesia is not necessary and it is performed in the doctor's office. Sometimes the examination is done under general anesthesia in very sensitive subjects or if 12 or even 16 biopsies are needed. The samples are then examined under a microscope.

Since there is a risk of infection, an antibiotic will be systematically prescribed before the examination. All anticoagulant and aspirin based treatments must be reported to the doctor so they can be stopped before the examination.

Patients need to check their temperature on the days following the biopsy, traces of blood may appear in the urine, sperm and bowel movements, which are not cause for alarm. This may last for a few weeks, and sometimes continue for 2 to 3 weeks.

CONCLUSION

Understanding prostate disorders is not always easy, basically they can be summarized as follows:
• a benign hypertrophy without symptoms does not need to be treated;
• and an early cancer without symptoms needs total removal of the prostate.

This conclusion is extremely simplified, but if a whole book was necessary to reach these two short sentences, it is because men and their partners ask themselves many questions about this little gland weighing just 15 grams (1/2 ounce), located at an important urinary and genital region, which can affect the image of male virility.

If these few pages make it possible to answer your questions, get you to eat a more balanced diet and fear prostate disease less, which is still a taboo subject, you'll be more likely to speak freely about it with your doctor or urologist because you'll know there are answers and solutions and this book will have fulfilled its modest function.

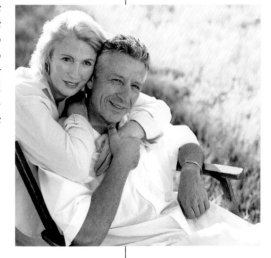

GLOSSARY

Antioxidant: substance capable of preventing, reducing or repairing damage caused by free radicals. An antioxidant can decrease or prevent cell oxidation.

Tranquilizer: a medicine used to fight anxiety.

Renal pelvis: A urine collecting funnel at the outlet of the kidneys situated between the calices and ureters.

Biopsy: removal of a small amount of tissue (sample) to be examined by an anatomical-pathologist doctor for diagnostic purposes

Renal calix: Urine collector tubes located between the kidneys taking urine to the renal pelvis.

Vas deferens: duct taking the sperm from the epididymis to the prostate.

Subpubic catheter: small drain perforating the skin below the pubis, to remove retention from the bladder when a catheterization is impossible.

Chemotherapy: treatment using medical substances to treat cancer; called cancer chemotherapy when cytotoxic drugs are used which destroy diseased cells. Given by IV, it makes it possible to treat the entire organism.

Celoscope: examination of the abdominal cavity with a optical fiber instrument introduced through a small cut in the skin. Other orifices can be used to introduce surgical instruments and this is referred to as celoscope surgery.

Cystoscopy : endoscopic examination of the bladder with a rigid instrument.

Detrusor: a bladder muscle, its contraction causes urination.

Dysuria: difficulty in urinating. The stream is weak.

Epididymis: duct taking the sperm from the testis to the vas deferens.

Fiberscopy: endoscopic examination using a flexible instrument, with optical fibers, much thinner than older rigid instruments. This is referred to as bladder fiberscopy for the bladder.

BPH: benign hypertrophy or hyperplasia of the prostate.

Hematuria: presence of blood in the urine.

Hematospermia: traces of blood in the sperm.

Hyperplasia: excessive development of tissue or an organ. Synonym: hypertrophy.

Metastasis: localization of cancer cells in another organ than the one where they originated.

Phlebitis: formation of a clot inside a vein sometimes associated with an inflammation of the vein wall. Phlebitis is often localized in the legs and the greatest risk is pulmonary embolism which can be fatal.

Pollakiuria: a need to urinate frequently.

PSA (Prostate Specific Antigen): plasma marker, its level is used to diagnose prostate diseases.

Spinal anesthesia: anesthesia of the lower part of the body by injection into the spine.

Septicemia: invasion of bacteria from an infected site in the blood stream, resulting in spiking temperature, chills, may be fatal due to cardio-respiratory system failure.

Stenosis: narrowing of a duct or vessel. In the case of the urethra, this may occur after infections, urethral catheter or an operation through the urethra.

Sclerosis: fibrous hardening, caused by scarring of an operated site often associated with narrowing of the area.

Ureter: duct taking urine from the renal pelvis to the bladder.

Urethra: Canal through which urine from the bladder is discharged to the exterior.

BIBLIOGRAPHY

Studies

Bent S : *Saw palmetto for benign prostatic hyperplasia.* N Engl J Med. 2006 Feb 9;354(6):557-66

Carbin E : *Treatment by curbicin in benign prostatic hyperplasia,* Swed J Biol Med 1989 ; 2 : 7-9.

Carbin E : *Treatment of benign prostatic hyperplasia with phytosterols,* British Journal of Urology 1990 ; 66 : 639-641.

Chan J : *Dairy products, calcium, and prostate cancer risk in the Physicians' Health Study.* American Journal of Clinical Nutrition 2001 ; 74 (4) : 549-554.

Clark L : *Decreased incidence of prostate cancer with selenium supplementation: results of a double-blind cancer prevention trial.* British Journal of Urology 1998 ; 81 (5) :730-734.

Demark-Wahnefried W. : *Pilot study of dietary fat restriction and flaxseed supplementation in men with prostate cancer before surgery : exploring the effects on hormonal levels, prostate-specific antigen and histopathologic features.* Urology 2001, 58(1) : 47-52.

Dutkiewicz S : *Usefulness of Cernilton in the treatment of benign prostatic hyperplasia.* International Urology and Nephrology 1996 ; 28 (1) : 49-53.

Gerber GS : *Randomized, double-blind, placebo controlled trial of saw palmetto in men with lower urinary tract symptoms.* The Journal of Urology 2001 ; 58 (6) : 960-964.

Giovannucci E : *A prospective study of dietary fat and risk of prostate cancer.* Journal of the National Cancer Institute 1993 ; 85 (19) :1571-1579.

Giovannucci E : *Obesity and benign prostatic hyperplasia.* American Journal of Epidemiology 1994 ; 140 (11) : 989-1002.

Giovannucci E : *Intake of carotenoids and retinol in relation to risk of prostate cancer.* Journal of the National Cancer Institute 1995 ; 87 (23) :1767-76.

Hanchette C : *Geographic patterns of prostate cancer mortality. Evidence for a protective effect of ultraviolet radiation.* Cancer 1992 ; 70 (12) : 2861-2869.

Heinonen P : *Prostate cancer and supplementation with alpha-tocopherol and beta-carotene: incidence and mortality in a controlled trial.* Journal of the National Cancer Institute 1998 ; 90 (6) : 440-446.

Hsing A : *Allium Vegetables and Risk of Prostate Cancer: A Population-Based Study.* Journal of the National Cancer Institute 2002, 94(21) : 1648-1651.

Hussain M : *Soy isoflavones in the treatment of prostate cancer.* 4th International Soy Symposium 2001.

Jenkins D : *Soy consumption and phytoestrogens: effect on serum prostate specific antigen when blood lipids and oxidized low-density lipoprotein are reduced in hyperlipidemic men.* Journal of Urology 2003 ; 169 (2) : 507-11.

Kirby R : *Efficacy and tolerability of doxazosin and finasteride, alone or in combination, in treatment of symptomatic benign prostatic hyperplasia: the Prospective European Doxazosin and Combination Therapy (PREDICT) trial.* Urology 2003 Jan ; 61(1):119-126.

Kristal R : *Vitamin and mineral supplement use is associated with reduced risk of prostate cancer.* Cancer Epidemiology Biomarkers & Prevention 1999 (10) : 887-892.

Kucuk O : *Effects of lycopene supplementation in patients with localized prostate cancer.* Experimental Biology and Medicine 2002 ; 227 (10) : 881-885.

Kushi L & Giovannucci E : *Dietary fat and cancer.* American Journal of Medicine 2002 ; 113 Suppl 9B : 63S-70S.

Metzker H : *Wirksamkeit eines Sabal-Urtica-kombinationspraparates bei der behandlung der benignen prostatahyperplasie (BPH).* Urologe 1996 ; 36 (4) : 292-300. Étude mentionnée et détaillée dans : Natural Standard (Ed). Herbs & Supplements - Saw palmetto, Nature Medicine Quality Standard. [Consulté le 6 janvier 2003]. www.naturalstandard.com

Mc Connel JD : *The Long term effects of medical therapy on the progression of BPH : results from the MTOPS trial.* Journal of Urology 2002; 167 (suppl) : 1042.

Michaud S : *A prospective study on intake of animal products and risk of prostate cancer.* Cancer Causes & Control 2001 ; 12 (6) :557-567.

Platz A : *Physical activity and benign prostatic hyperplasia.* Archives of Internal Medicine 1998 ; 158 (21) : 2349-2356.

Suzuki S : *Intakes of energy and macronutrients and the risk of benign prostatic hyperplasia.* American Journal of Clinical Nutrition 2002, 75 (4) : 689-697.

Terry P : *Fatty fish consumption and risk of prostate cancer.* The Lancet 2001 ; 357 (9270) : 1764-1766.

Uzzo G : *Zinc Inhibits Nuclear Factor-kappaB Activation and Sensitizes Prostate Cancer Cells to Cytotoxic Agents.* Clinical Cancer Research 2002 ; 8 (11) : 3579-3583.

Wilt J : *Beta-sitosterol for the treatment of benign prostatic hyperplasia: a systematic review.* British Journal of Urology 1999 ; 83 (9) : 976-983.

Wilt T : *Pygeum africanum for benign prostatic hyperplasia.* Cochrane Database of Systematic Reviews 2002 ; (1) : CD001044.

Zhou J : *Soy phytochemicals and tea bioactive components synergistically inhibit androgen-sensitive human prostate tumors in mice.* The Journal of Nutrition 2003 ; 133 (2) : 516-521.

Zhu S : *Waist circumference and obesity-associated risk factors among whites in the third National Health and Nutrition Examination Survey: clinical action thresholds.* American Journal of Clinical Nutrition 2002, 76 (4) : 743-749.

Publications :

Grosclaude P : *Cancer de la prostate. In : Alimentation et cancer – Evaluation des données scientifiques.* CNERNA et CNRS. Tec&Doc. 1996.

Food, Nutrition and the Prevention of Cancer : a global perspective. World Cancer research Fund / American Institute for Cancer Research. 1997 (pp. 310-323).

Bertrand Guillonneau et Guy Vallancien : *UROLOGIE-* InterMed. Doin Editeurs, Paris, 1999.

Vincent Ravery : *Cancer de la Prostate.* Springer Verlag France, Paris, 2002.

Patrice Pfeifer : *La prostate au quotidien.* Odile Jacob, 1999.

In our collection Alpen Éditions:

-The Omega-3 Answer

-Living with a Hyperactive Child

-All About the Prostate

-The French Paradox

-The XXL Syndrome

with Michel Montignac:

-Eat Yourself Slim

-The Montignac Diet Cookbook

-The French GI Diet

-Glycemic Index Diet

www.alpen.mc